GOUT
The Indian Scenario

GOUT
The Indian Scenario

Editors

Sachin Yashwant Kale MS(Orthopedics)
D Ortho FCPS Fellowship in Arthroplasty
Professor and Head of Unit
Department of Orthopedics
Dr DY Patil School of Medicine
Consultant Orthopedic Surgeon
Apollo Hospital, Belapur
Fortis Hiranandani Hospital, Vashi,
Navi Mumbai, Maharashtra, India

Shivam Mehra MBBS MS(Orthopedics)
Fellowship in Pediatric Upper Limb
Deformity Correction' from
National Center for Child Health and
Development, Tokyo, Japan
Short-term Fellowship in Deformity
Correction and Limb Lengthening from
Paley's Institute, Florida
Consultant, Department of Orthopedics
Mehra Hospital and Research Institute
Lucknow, Uttar Pradesh, India

Co-Editors

Nindiya Kapoor Mehra MTech
Biotechnology(IIT Kanpur)
Executive Management Course in Hospital
Management(IIM Ahmedabad)
Research and Administration Head
Mehra Hospital and Research Institute
Lucknow, Uttar Pradesh, India

Vishal Kumar MS DNB FRCS
Professor (Additional)
Department of Orthopedics
PGIMER
Chandigarh, India

Sub-Editors

Kamal Mehra
Bharat Veer Manchanda
Pramod Bhor

Arvind J Vatkar
Smruti Sachin Kale

Foreword
Prakash Samant

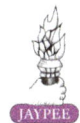

JAYPEE BROTHERS MEDICAL PUBLISHERS
The Health Sciences Publisher
New Delhi | London

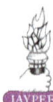 **Jaypee Brothers Medical Publishers (P) Ltd**

Headquarters
EMCA House
23/23-B, Ansari Road, Daryaganj
New Delhi 110 002, India
Landline: +91-11-23272143
 +91-11-23272703, +91-11-23282021
+91-11-23245672
E-mail: jaypee@jaypeebrothers.com

Corporate Office
Jaypee Brothers Medical Publishers (P) Ltd
4838/24, Ansari Road, Daryaganj
New Delhi 110 002, India
Phone: +91-11-43574357
Fax: +91-11-43574314
E-mail: jaypee@jaypeebrothers.com

Overseas Office
JP Medical Ltd.
83, Victoria Street, London
SW1H 0HW (UK)
Phone: +44-20 3170 8910
E-mail: info@jpmedpub.com

EU GPSR Authorised Representative
Logos Europe, 9 rue Nicolas Poussin
17000, La Rochelle, France
Phone: +33 (0) 6 67 93 73 78
E-mail: Contact@logoseurope.eu

Website: www.jaypeebrothers.com

Website: www.jaypeedigital.com

© 2025, Jaypee Brothers Medical Publishers

The views and opinions expressed in this book are solely those of the original contributor(s)/author(s) and do not necessarily represent those of editor(s) or publisher of the book.

All rights reserved. No part of this publication may be reproduced, stored or transmitted in any form or by any means, electronic, mechanical, photocopying, recording or otherwise, without the prior permission in writing of the publishers.

All brand names and product names used in this book are trade names, service marks, trademarks or registered trademarks of their respective owners. The publisher is not associated with any product or vendor mentioned in this book.

Medical knowledge and practice change constantly. This book is designed to provide accurate, authoritative information about the subject matter in question. However, readers are advised to check the most current information available on procedures included and check information from the manufacturer of each product to be administered, to verify the recommended dose, formula, method and duration of administration, adverse effects and contraindications. It is the responsibility of the practitioner to take all appropriate safety precautions. Neither the publisher nor the author(s)/editor(s) assume any liability for any injury and/or damage to persons or property arising from or related to use of material in this book.

This book is sold on the understanding that the publisher is not engaged in providing professional medical services. If such advice or services are required, the services of a competent medical professional should be sought.

Every effort has been made where necessary to contact holders of copyright to obtain permission to reproduce copyright material. If any have been inadvertently overlooked, the publisher will be pleased to make the necessary arrangements at the first opportunity.

Inquiries for bulk sales may be solicited at: jaypee@jaypeebrothers.com

GOUT: The Indian Scenario / **Sachin Yashwant Kale, Shivam Mehra**

First Edition: 2025

ISBN: 978-93-6616-865-4

Contributors

Aditya Gupta MS
Senior Resident
Department of Orthopedics
PGIMER
Chandigarh, India

Arvind J Vatkar
MS(Orthopedics) AFIH MCh Spine
Surgery (Edgehill University, UK)
Advanced Spine Surgery Fellowship
(Nottingham UK)
Assistant Professor
Department of Orthopedics
MGM Medical College
(Proposed), Nerul, Navi Mumbai
Consultant Orthopedic Spine
Surgeon Apollo Hospital,
Belapur
Fortis Hiranandani Hospital
Vashi, Navi Mumbai
Maharashtra, India

Bharat Veer Manchanda
MBBS MD(Medicine) Postdoctoral
Fellowship Rheumatology (CRD
Pune)
Owner and Consultant
Rheumatologist
Arthritis & Breast Care Centre
Kurukshetra, Haryana
Visiting Rheumatologist
Amritdhara Hospital, Karnal,
Haryana Baweja Hospital
Ambala, Haryana, India

Kamal Mehra MBBS D Ortho
(Surgery) MS(Orthopedics)
Johnson & Johnson Fellowship
in Joint Replacement
Ex-President, Lucknow
Orthopaedic Club
Director and Senior Consultant
Mehra Hospital and Research
Institute
Lucknow, Uttar Pradesh, India

Nindiya Kapoor Mehra MTech
Biotechnology(IIT Kanpur)
Executive Management Course
in Hospital Management(IIM
Ahmedabad)
Research and Administration
Head
Mehra Hospital and Research
Institute
Lucknow, Uttar Pradesh, India

Prakash Samant MBBS
MS(Orthopedics)
Professor and Head
Department of Orthopedics
Dr DY Patil School of Medicine
Navi Mumbai, Maharashtra, India

Pramod Bhor MBBS
MS(Orthopedics)
Director
Department of Orthopedics
Fortis Hiranandani Hospital
Navi Mumbai, Maharashtra, India

Contributors

Sachin Yashwant Kale
MS(Orthopedics) D Ortho FCPS
Fellowship in Arthroplasty
Professor and Head of Unit
Department of Orthopedics
Dr DY Patil School of Medicine
Consultant Orthopedic Surgeon
Apollo Hospital, Belapur
Fortis Hiranandani Hospital
Vashi, Navi Mumbai,
Maharashtra, India

Sachiti Sachin Kale
MBBS(Second Year)
Lokmanya Tilak Medical College
and Sion Hospital
Mumbai, Maharashtra, India

Shivam Mehra MBBS
MS(Orthopedics)
Fellowship in Pediatric Upper
Limb Deformity Correction'
from National Center for Child
Health and Development
Tokyo, Japan
Short-term Fellowship in
Deformity Correction and Limb
Lengthening from Paley's
Institute, Florida
Consultant
Department of Orthopedics
Mehra Hospital and Research
Institute
Lucknow, Uttar Pradesh, India

Smruti Sachin Kale MBBS DGO
Owner Sachi Hospital
Department of Obstetrician and
Gynecologist
Sachi Hospital, Airoli,
Navi Mumbai, Maharashtra,
India

Sumedha Shinde MBBS
MD(Pathology)
Assistant Professor
Department of Transfusion
Medicine, Sir JJ Blood Centre,
Grant Government Medical
College
Mumbai, Maharashtra, India

Sunil Shetty MBBS
MS(Orthopedics)
Professor
Department of Orthopedics
Dr DY Patil School of Medicine
Navi Mumbai, Maharashtra,
India

Vishal Kumar MS DNB FRCS
Professor (Additional)
Department of Orthopedics
PGIMER
Chandigarh, India

Foreword

The rising prevalence of hyperuricemia and gout in India underscores the urgent need for comprehensive resources tailored to the unique demographic and environmental factors influencing the Indian population. This handbook, *"Gout: The Indian Scenario"*, serves as a pivotal guide for healthcare professionals, researchers, and students seeking to understand and manage elevated uric acid levels and gout within the Indian context.

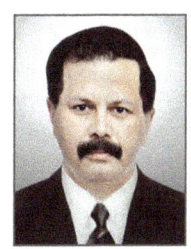

Gout, often dismissed as a disease of indulgence, is a complex condition influenced by a myriad of genetic, environmental, and lifestyle factors. In India, the intersection of traditional dietary habits, genetic predispositions, and rapidly changing lifestyles has resulted in an increase in gout cases. This handbook meticulously explores these nuances, providing a detailed analysis and practical insights into the management of gout specific to Indian communities.

The chapters in this handbook are authored by a distinguished panel of experts who bring a wealth of knowledge and clinical experience. Each chapter delves into critical aspects of gout and hyperuricemia, offering evidence-based information and recommendations.

- Chapter 1 lays the foundation with a comprehensive introduction to hyperuricemia and gout, discussing the biochemical underpinnings, symptoms, diagnosis, and treatment strategies.
- Chapter 2 focuses on the metabolism of uric acid, elucidating the differences between normal and hyperuricemic states.
- Chapter 3 presents findings from a multicentric study on Indian communities, shedding light on the epidemiology and demographic factors affecting uric acid levels.

- Chapter 4 examines the correlation between menopause and increased uric acid levels, providing crucial insights into managing gout in postmenopausal women.
- Chapter 5 discusses the application of local heat and massage in gout-affected joints, offering practical advice on alternative therapies.
- Chapter 6 compares the impact of alcohol and protein-rich foods on gout, guiding dietary strategies for effective management.
- Chapter 7 addresses the diagnostic challenges of idiopathic retrocalcaneal pain and heel pain in the context of gout.
- Chapter 8 explores the occurrence and management of gout during pregnancy, highlighting its impact on maternal and fetal health.
- Chapter 9 focuses on gout in the spine, detailing its pathophysiology, clinical manifestations, and management strategies.
- Chapter 10 provides a concise list of do's and don'ts, along with lifestyle changes to manage and prevent gout.
- Chapter 11 discusses the complex challenges of managing gout in India, emphasizing a holistic approach.
- Chapter 12 offers a detailed review of various antigout drugs and their efficacy in the Indian context.

This handbook is the result of the collaborative efforts of a team of esteemed editors and co-editors who have meticulously curated and compiled the latest research and clinical insights into gout and hyperuricemia.

Editors:

Sachin Yashwant Kale is a renowned expert in the field of orthopedics. He has made significant contributions to the understanding and management of gout in the Indian population. His clinical expertise and research acumen have been instrumental in shaping the content of this handbook.

Shivam Mehra is an accomplished orthopedic surgeon with a deep understanding of metabolic disorders. He has played a crucial role in providing a comprehensive perspective on gout and its management. His dedication to patient care and research excellence is reflected throughout this book.

Co-Editors:

Nindiya Kapoor Mehra: With a background in medical research, tissue engineering, drug discovery in autoimmune diseases and biosimilars, Mrs Mehra has contributed her expertise in epidemiology and data analysis, ensuring that the handbook is grounded in robust scientific evidence. Her insights into the genetic and environmental factors affecting uric acid levels have added a valuable dimension to this work.

Vishal Kumar is a distinguished surgeon and researcher. His contributions to this handbook include detailed explorations of diagnostic and therapeutic strategies for gout. His commitment to advancing medical knowledge and improving patient outcomes is evident in the depth and clarity of the content presented.

In conclusion, *"Gout: The Indian Scenario"* is an indispensable resource that addresses the multifaceted challenges of managing gout in India. It provides a thorough understanding of the disease, its implications, and practical approaches to treatment, making it a valuable tool for improving patient outcomes. We hope that this handbook will inspire further research and foster a deeper understanding of gout within the Indian Medical Community.

Prakash Samant
MBBS MS(Orthopedics)
Professor and Head
Department of Orthopedics
Dr DY Patil School of Medicine
Navi Mumbai, Maharashtra, India

Preface

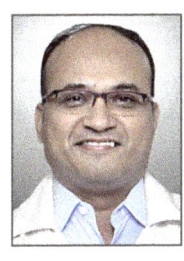

In recent years, the prevalence of gout and hyperuricemia has risen significantly, particularly in India. Despite its historical association with affluence, gout is now increasingly affecting diverse populations, emphasizing the need for a clearer understanding of this complex condition. This handbook, titled *"Gout: The Indian Scenario,"* aims to provide a comprehensive exploration of elevated uric acid levels and gout within the sociocultural context of India.

This handbook features contributions from a multidisciplinary team of experts who bring their extensive knowledge and clinical experience to light. Each chapter is meticulously crafted to address different facets of gout, ranging from its biochemical and metabolic origins to its social impact and management strategies tailored for the Indian demographic. Our contributors—recognized professionals in their fields—have endeavored to present evidence-based information while also considering cultural factors that influence dietary and lifestyle choices.

Chapter titles encompass critical areas of study, including the metabolism of uric acid, the rising incidence of gout post menopause, the role of dietary habits, and the implications of gout during pregnancy. Notably, this handbook delves into specific Indian communities, providing insights through data-driven analyses from multicentric studies, allowing for targeted discussions reflecting the unique challenges faced in our country.

As we explore the problem of gout from various perspectives, it is important to highlight the need for holistic approaches to treatment and management. The insights shared herein are designed to empower healthcare professionals, researchers, and patients alike with the knowledge necessary to improve health outcomes and enhance the quality of life for those affected by gout.

We sincerely hope that this handbook will serve as a valuable resource for readers, fostering a deeper understanding of gout and highlighting the importance of patient education, compliance, and community awareness in combating this disease.

Thank you for joining us on this journey to better understand *"Gout: The Indian Scenario."* We wish you a fruitful and enlightening reading experience!

Sachin Yashwant Kale

Preface

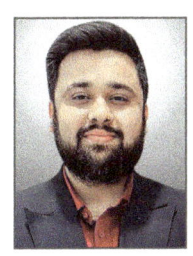

Gout is the most prevalent form of inflammatory arthritis in adults globally. It disproportionately affects men, the elderly, and racial/ethnic minorities. Gout commonly co-exists with other health conditions, which complicates its management and adds to the overall burden of the disease. In India, the prevalence of gout has been increasing due to lifestyle changes, increased consumption of purine-rich foods, and higher rates of obesity and metabolic syndrome.

The prevalence of hyperuricemia in the Indian population has been estimated to range from 20 to 25% in various studies and approximately 1–2% of the adult Indian population being affected by gout. Having said that, there is scarce data on the manifestation of hyperuricemia and gout when we consider factors such as regional differences, urban versus rural population, and religion and community-based differences.

This book, *"Gout: The Indian Scenario"*, is a practical handbook on the prevalence of elevated uric acid levels and gout in the Indian perspective. The book aims to provide a comprehensive overview of hyperuricemia and gout by addressing relevant and practical details. Our objective is to present a thorough understanding of this disease through the lens of current evidence and clinical experience.

The book provides a deeper understanding of gout and hyperuricemia by discussing aspects in pregnancy, menopause, manifestation in spine, the do's and don'ts, and much more. Further, our study conducted at Dr DY Patil Medical College and Hospital forms the central pillar of this book. It is a multicentric study done in more than 10,000 patients over a span of 3 years to provide an estimate on the levels of uric acid in different religious

Indian communities, that is, Hindu, Muslim, Sikh, and Christians. The results of the study highlight clear variations in uric acid levels based on various factors that differ in these communities. Hence, the need for such studies is of utmost importance to guide better treatment for hyperuricemia and gout.

Addressing gout in India requires a multifaceted approach involving dietary and lifestyle changes, effective medical treatment, public health awareness, and improved healthcare access. By tackling the risk factors and promoting healthy living, the burden of gout can be significantly reduced.

We hope this book serves as a valuable resource for orthopedic surgeons, rheumatologists, researchers, and healthcare professionals involved in the management of hyperuricemia and gout. By sharing our experience and the broader evidence base, we aim to enhance understanding and improve patient outcomes for this challenging disease.

Shivam Mehra

Preface

Gout, once known as the "disease of kings," has evolved into a common and significant health concern affecting millions of people worldwide, including in India. With its sharp, sudden attacks of pain and its potential to cause chronic disability, gout stands as a poignant reminder of the intricate relationship between our lifestyle choices, dietary habits, and overall health.

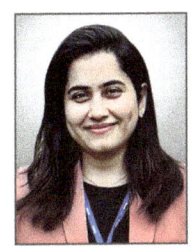

This book is born out of a necessity to provide a comprehensive understanding of gout, particularly within the Indian context. As the prevalence of gout rises in tandem with lifestyle changes, it becomes imperative to disseminate accurate information and practical advice to both healthcare providers and the general public. Our aim is to bridge the knowledge gap, offering insights into the causes, symptoms, diagnosis, treatment, and management of gout.

We delve into the introduction and metabolism of uric acid, the molecule responsible for hyperuricemia, gout and associated metabolic disorders. Understanding its role in the body provides valuable context for appreciating the modern advancements in its diagnosis and treatment. The book then transitions into a detailed exploration of the pathophysiology of gout, shedding light on how elevated uric acid levels lead to the formation of painful urate crystals in the joints.

One of the key focuses of this book is the impact of diet and lifestyle on gout. Traditional Indian diets, rich in purine-containing foods, coupled with modern sedentary lifestyles, have contributed to the rising incidence of this condition. We discuss the role of dietary modifications, weight management, and other lifestyle changes in preventing and managing gout. Our goal is to empower readers with practical, actionable advice that can help mitigate the risk of gout attacks and improve the overall quality of life.

Additionally, this book addresses the medical management of gout, including both acute and long-term treatment strategies. We provide an overview of the medications commonly used, their mechanisms of action, and potential side effects. Understanding the full spectrum of treatment options allows patients and healthcare providers to make informed decisions tailored to individual needs.

Public health initiatives and research are also pivotal in the fight against gout. We highlight the importance of awareness campaigns, early diagnosis, and continuous research to develop better treatment modalities. By staying informed about the latest advancements and best practices, we can collectively work toward reducing the burden of gout in our society.

This book is a collaborative effort, drawing on the expertise of leading rheumatologists, orthopedists, and health professionals. We have strived to present complex medical information in an accessible and engaging manner, ensuring that this book serves as a valuable resource for both healthcare providers and patients alike.

In conclusion, we hope this book serves as a comprehensive guide to understanding, managing, and preventing gout. By fostering a deeper understanding of this condition, we can work toward a future where gout is no longer a debilitating disease but a manageable aspect of life.

Thank you for embarking on this journey with us!

Nindiya Kapoor Mehra

Preface

Gout is a common clinical entity in day-to-day practice of medical professionals across specialties, but the absence of a single guidebook on the shelves of the clinicians made us compose this compendium. This handbook is all the more easy to carry, read, and refer. It gives a comprehensive in-depth coverage of gout and related disorders, more so in context with the Indian scenario but 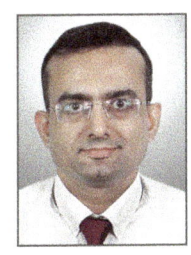 a guide to read and refer across the globe. This is an important stakeholder on shelves for gout for both undergraduate and postgraduate students as well as for teachers, researchers, and clinicians across specialties.

This guidebook vividly covers the relevant expert guidance in a very user-friendly format on diet and lifestyle modifications and preventive measures to avert gout and related hyperuricemic disorders. It has a special focus on the recent research and advancement in literature related to the gout and related disorders.

Gout can present with diverse clinical presentations, making it challenging to diagnose and manage at times. Over the past many years, various modalities of diagnosis and treatment have been investigated and evolved including lifestyle modifications, pharmacotherapy, and surgery. This book aims to address an overview of gout and related disorders, highlight and comment on diverse presentations and plausible diagnostic challenges, and elaborate on the management options. It also covers recent advances in diagnostic modalities and surgical management of the disease with a vision on the scope of possible research in future. This book is written by authoritative authors across the country with several years of successful experience in treating a myriad of patients afflicted with gout and related disorders.

We wish this composed compendium serves its goal of being the guiding textbook and reference work on gout.

Thank you team Jaypee Brothers Medical Publishers for pairing with us to complete the paint on the picture of gout!

Vishal Kumar

Acknowledgments

We, the editorial team members, take this privileged opportunity to thank and congratulate all the gifted authors for coming out with this compendium on Gout, a common clinical entity which we all come across in our day-to-day practice. The authors of this book are across walls and boundaries with immense knowledge and experience in practice for this clinical condition. The compliance of the authors to the timeline for their designated chapters and mutual discussions, including comments, criticism, and appreciation on the different chapters of the book, among us while composing the assigned compendium have transformed this book into a reference book on "Gout" for the interested readers. The mutual cooperation and cohesion among the editorial teammates has been phenomenal to bring out this book well within the stipulated time.

We also express our overwhelming gratitude to our family members, who are the immediate ones to bear the pain of our absence due to involvement in preparing this academic treatise. Their support, care, patience, and motivation have been exceptional all throughout.

We are deeply grateful to Shri Jitendar P Vij (Group Chairman), Mr Ankit Vij (Managing Director), Mr MS Mani (Group President), Ms Chetna Malhotra (Senior Director—Professional Publishing, Marketing, and Business Development), Ms Pooja Bhandari [Director—Production (Books and Journals)], and Mr Akhilesh Saxena (Publishing Coordinator), M/s Jaypee Brothers Medical Publishers (P) Ltd, New Delhi, India, for their professional support and dedication to bringing this book to life. Their team has been phenomenal for being there for us round the clock with their platform and commitment to enhance and propagate scientific learning and knowledge.

We extend our heartfelt gratitude to our friends and colleagues who have time and again helped us in shaping the book in the form it is today by their insights, wisdom, and encouragement.

Patients are the pillars of our clinics, research, and academics. Hence, the editors and authors of this book take a bow for the patience and perseverance of our patients, without whom we cannot even dream of this journey.

Finally, it is the readers whose enthusiasm, encouragement, and zeal to read and learn keep our spirits of writing high, and we are really indebted to them.

Hope we are able to deliver up to the expectations of readers.

Thank you Almighty for making us the blessed and the privileged!

The Editorial Team

Contents

1. **Introduction to Hyperuricemia and Gout**   1
   *Shivam Mehra, Kamal Mehra, Nindiya Kapoor Mehra,
   Bharat Veer Manchanda, Arvind J Vatkar*

2. **Metabolism of Uric Acid**   14
   *Nindiya Kapoor Mehra, Shivam Mehra,
   Sumedha Shinde, Sachiti Sachin Kale*

3. **Indian Communities and their Effect on Elevated Uric Acid Levels: A Multicentric Study**   25
   *Sachin Yaswant Kale, Kamal Mehra, Shivam Mehra,
   Nindiya Kapoor Mehra, Bharat Veer Manchanda*

4. **Increase in Incidence of Uric Acid Levels and Gout Postmenopause**   33
   *Kamal Mehra, Nindiya Kapoor Mehra, Shivam Mehra,
   Smruti Sachin Kale*

5. **Application of Local Heat and Massage in Gout-affected Joints**   43
   *Shivam Mehra, Kamal Mehra, Prakash Samant,
   Sachin Yaswant Kale, Pramod Bhor*

6. **Who is the Biggest Culprit for Gout: Alcohol or Protein-rich Foods or Both?**   49
   Aditya Gupta, Vishal Kumar

7. **Idiopathic Retrocalcaneal Pain and Heel Pain: Is it Gout?**   57
   *Prakash Samant, Arvind J Vatkar, Sachin Yaswant Kale,
   Shivam Mehra, Sunil Shetty, Pramod Bhor*

8. **Gout in Pregnancy**   68
   *Smruti Sachin Kale, Sumedha Shinde,
   Nindiya Kapoor Mehra, Sachiti Sachin Kale*

9. **Gout in Spine** — 77
 Arvind J Vatkar, Sachin Yashwant Kale, Vishal Kumar, Aditya Gupta

10. **Gout: The Do's and Don'ts** — 85
 Vishal Kumar, Shivam Mehra, Kamal Mehra, Sunil Shetty

11. **Gout: The Unsatisfied Disease—A Complex Challenge in the Indian Scenario** — 96
 Sachin Yashwant Kale, Arvind J Vatkar, Shivam Mehra

12. **Topiroxostat, Febuxostat, Allopurinol, Colchicine, and Probenecid: A Review in Indian Communities** — 101
 Bharat Veer Manchanda, Nindiya Kapoor Mehra, Shivam Mehra

Summary and Key Takeaways — *127*

Index — *129*

CHAPTER 1

Introduction to Hyperuricemia and Gout

Shivam Mehra, Kamal Mehra, Nindiya Kapoor Mehra, Bharat Veer Manchanda, Arvind J Vatkar

INTRODUCTION

Uric acid is a chemical molecule produced when the body breaks down purines. Purines are chemical substances contained in DNA and RNA that are necessary for cell function and play an important role in biological processes such as nucleotide synthesis. They have a two-ring structure and are often found in adenine and guanine with their chemical formulae of $C_5H_5N_5$ and $C_5H_5N_5O$, respectively. Purines are present in a variety of foods, with the highest concentrations found in organ meats, shellfish, and vegetables such as asparagus, cauliflower, spinach, mushrooms, and green peas.

Uric acid is an organic compound that contains carbon (C), hydrogen (H), nitrogen (N), and oxygen (O) atoms. The molecular formula is $C_5H_4N_4O_3$, and its structure consists of a fused ring system with nitrogen atoms **(Fig. 1)**.

Uric acid was first discovered in the late 18th century. Swedish scientist Carl Wilhelm Scheele discovered uric acid in 1776 while researching kidney stones. Scientists like Sir Archibald Garrod conducted more studies in the 19th century to better understand its involvement in gout and other metabolic illnesses.

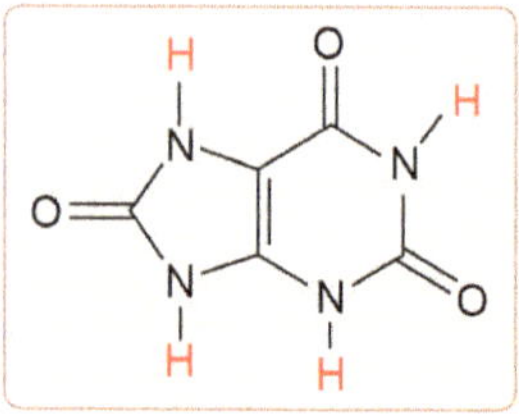

Fig. 1: Molecular structure of uric acid.

URIC ACID, HYPERURICEMIA, AND GOUT

Uric acid is the result of extrinsic pool of purines and intrinsic purine metabolism in humans and higher primates. In all other mammals, the enzyme uricase converts uric acid to allantoin that gets eliminated through urine. The metabolism and production of uric acid involve processes that depend on multiple factors regulating its production in the liver and excretion by the gut and kidneys. Uric acid predominantly exists as urate, that is, in its salt form. The rise in the urate concentration in blood leads to the formation of uric acid crystals. Since it has a low water solubility (solubility limit in blood being 6.8 mg/dL in humans), higher levels of uric acid (>6.8 mg/dL) result in the formation of monosodium urate crystals (MSU).

Higher uric acid levels or hyperuricemia is a product of more uric acid production, dysfunctional renal excretion, or a combination of both. Hyperuricemia leads to deposition of urate crystals in the joints and kidneys. Increasing evidence suggests the relationship of hyperuricemia with multiple conditions including gout, diabetes, hypertension, renal disease, metabolic syndrome, and cardiovascular disease.

Gout is a form of arthritis that is associated with hyperuricemia. It occurs when urate crystals, formed from excess uric acid, accumulate in the joints, causing inflammation, pain, and swelling. Gout typically affects the big toe but can also impact other joints such as the ankles, knees, elbows, wrists, and fingers.

The link between hyperuricemia and disease is the strongest for gout, a common rheumatic disease characterized by acute inflammatory arthritis. Around 8.3 million Americans are affected by gout. Although these numbers in India are not very clear. A study conducted in Bhigwan Village of India estimated a prevalence of 0.12% according to the International League of Nations Against Rheumatism, Community Oriented Program for Control of Rheumatic Diseases (ILAR COPCORD). Another study revealed that 15.8% of affected patients are <30 years of age and urban Indian population has more presence compared to rural population.

FACTORS AFFECTING URIC ACID LEVELS: GENETIC AND ENVIRONMENTAL FACTORS

The cause of high uric acid level could be genetic or due to environmental factors such as diet and health. The correlation of diet with uric acid levels has not been fully understood, however, purine-rich foods such as meat (for example, red meat, bacon, pork, and mutton) and seafood have been suggested to increase uric acid levels. Choi and coworkers conducted a study for the association of gout with purine-rich foods, protein intake, and dairy intake. During 12 years of follow-up amongst 47,120 men that had no history of gout at baseline, 730 new cases of gout were reported. The authors reported a 1.41-fold and 1.51-fold increase in the risk of gout with increased meat and seafood consumption, respectively. No increased risk was found with increase in total protein intake and purine-rich vegetables. The study also reported that the risk of gout was low with higher consumption of low-fat dairy products.

Alcohol intake particularly consumption of purine-rich alcoholic beverages like beer is associated with increased risk for hyperuricemia. In another study by Choi and Curhan including data from 14,809 participants (both men and women) in the Third National Health and Nutrition Examination Survey (NHANES), the authors documented that serum uric acid levels increased with increasing beer consumption followed by liquor intake (p values for trend < 0.001) whereas moderate wine drinking does not affect serum uric acid levels. Also, it has been shown that alcohol intake increases uric acid both by reducing urate excretion and increasing production.

Multiple reports have also been published on the association of cigarette smoking with uric acid levels. It is reported that there is an inverse relation between smoking and serum uric acid levels. A study conducted on 300 participants reported that plasma uric acid levels were significantly lower in smokers than in nonsmokers. However, another study on Japanese male working population showed that serum uric acid levels were more in ex-smokers followed by nonsmokers and then present smokers.Another major risk factor for hyperuricemia is sedentary lifestyle. It was shown in a study that participants who spent ≥10 h/day in sedentary behavior were more likely to have hyperuricemia than those who spent <5 h/day.

As external factors and lifestyle are risk parameters for hyperuricemia and since lifestyle choices vary amongst the different Indian communities, we sought to study the prevalence of hyperuricemia in these communities. Also, there is a dearth of large-scale data (in terms of gender, age, lifestyle, and community) on the prevalence of hyperuricemia in subjects amongst different community populations. In this book, we talk about a multicentric prospective study that was undertaken to determine the prevalence of hyperuricemia in subjects across four major communities.

Further, we also demonstrate our study that determined the association between increased uric acid levels and lifestyle of different communities.

CHAPTER 1: Introduction to Hyperuricemia and Gout

CAUSES OF HYPERURICEMIA AND GOUT

- *Diet*: High intake of purine-rich foods (red meat, seafood, and organ meats), alcohol, and sugary beverages
- *Genetics*: Family history of gout or hyperuricemia
- Gout, a condition characterized by elevated uric acid levels and urate crystal formation in joints, is largely influenced by genetics. Recent studies have identified several genetic variants linked to increased risk of gout, including SLC2A9, ABCG2, and SLC22A12, which regulate uric acid transport and excretion. A 2018 study highlighted the importance of genetic predisposition in gout, with certain alleles increasing the risk by affecting renal urate handling and promoting hyperuricemia. Another 2020 study highlighted the role of ABCG2 mutations in early-onset gout. Gout inheritance is complex, involving autosomal dominant and polygenic mechanisms. Families with a history of gout often show a higher prevalence, suggesting a hereditary component. Gene therapy for gout is still in its experimental stages, with researchers exploring the potential of CRISPR-Cas9 technology to correct specific genetic mutations associated with hyperuricemia.
- *Medical conditions*: Obesity, hypertension, kidney disease, diabetes, and metabolic syndrome.
- *Medications*: Certain drugs may exacerbate gout by raising uric acid levels via a variety of ways. Diuretics, such as thiazide and loop diuretics, impede kidney uric acid excretion, resulting in hyperuricemia. Low-dose aspirin reduces renal urate excretion and promotes uric acid retention. Immunosuppressants, such as cyclosporine, reduce renal urate production, which contributes to high uric acid levels. Niacin, which is used to treat cholesterol, may also raise uric acid levels by decreasing renal urate clearance. Gout may interact with drugs, necessitating dosage modifications. Understanding these interactions

is critical for healthcare practitioners seeking to optimize treatment methods for gout patients, ensuring successful management and reducing medication-related problems.

SYMPTOMS OF GOUT

- Sudden, intense joint pain
- Swelling and redness around the affected joint
- Warmth and tenderness in the joint
- Limited range of motion in the affected joint
- Acute gout is characterized by the rapid onset of intense pain, swelling, warmth, and redness in the afflicted joint, which often wakes patients from their sleep. The first episode normally peaks within 24 hours and may linger anywhere from a few days to a couple of weeks if not addressed. Podagra, a special word for gout affecting the big toe, is the most prevalent presentation in 50% of first-time gout attacks, producing severe pain and inflammation at the metatarsophalangeal joints. Other joints affected by gout include the ankles, knees, elbows, wrists, and fingers, which become painful, erythematous, and swollen, limiting mobility and quality of life.

DIAGNOSIS OF HYPERURICEMIA AND GOUT

- *Blood test*: Measures the level of uric acid in the blood.
- *Joint fluid test*: Checks for urate crystals in the synovial fluid.
- *Imaging*: X-rays, ultrasound, or CT scans to detect joint damage or crystal deposits. Gout X-rays are frequently seen later in the disease.

Signs include tophi are soft tissue opacities caused by the deposition of urate crystal. Ultrasound would show joint effusion which refers to an increase in joint fluid. "Rat bite" lesions are defined as periarticular or marginal erosions with overhanging borders. Well-defined sclerotic borders. Chronic

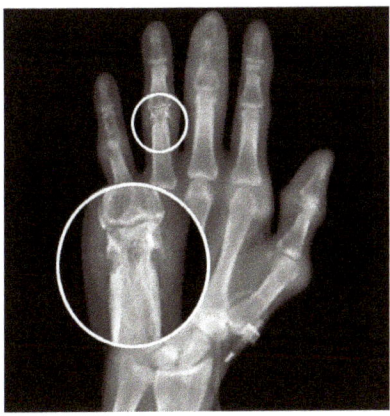

Fig. 2: Rat bite erosions seen in hand X-ray in gout.
Source: Gibson MC. Gout x ray. [online] Available from https://www.wikidoc.org/index.php/Gout_x_ray [Last accessed August, 2024].

joint space narrowing suggests cartilage deterioration. *Bone changes*—subchondral bone cysts and spurs may develop **(Fig. 2)**.

TREATMENT AND MANAGEMENT OF GOUT

- *Medications*:
  - *Nonsteroidal anti-inflammatory drugs (NSAIDs)*: To reduce inflammation and pain
  - *Colchicine*: To relieve acute gout attacks
  - *Corticosteroids*: To control severe inflammation
  - *Urate-lowering therapy*: Allopurinol or febuxostat to reduce uric acid levels.
- *Lifestyle changes*:
  - *Diet*: Reduce intake of purine-rich foods, alcohol, and sugary drinks.
  - *Hydration*: Drink plenty of water to help flush out uric acid.

- *Weight management*: Achieve and maintain a healthy weight.
  - *Exercise*: Regular physical activity to improve overall health.
- *Preventive measures*: Regular monitoring of uric acid levels and adherence to prescribed treatments to prevent recurrent gout attacks.

DIFFERENTIAL DIAGNOSIS

- *Pseudogout* (calcium pyrophosphate deposition disease) often affects bigger joints, such as the knee. Frequently has a more chronic course.

  Special tests include joint aspiration reveals calcium pyrophosphate crystals that are rhomboid-shaped and positively birefringent under polarized light **(Fig. 3)**.

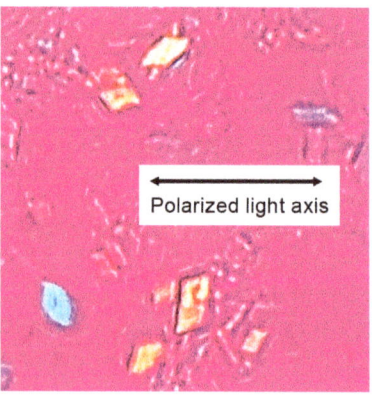

Fig. 3: Microscopy showing rhomboid shaped crystals in synovial fluid of pseudogout.
Source: Wikipedia. Calcium pyrophosphate dihydrate crystal deposition disease. [online] Available from https://en.wikipedia.org/wiki/Calcium_pyrophosphate_dihydrate_crystal_deposition_disease [Last accessed August, 2024].

- *Septic arthritis symptoms*: Severe pain, fever, and high white blood cell count. Affects every joint, but particularly the knee.

    Special tests include joint aspiration with a positive bacterial culture and an increased white blood cell count in synovial fluid. Gram staining of synovial fluid may reveal bacterial organisms.
- *Rheumatoid arthritis* symptoms include symmetric joint involvement, prolonged morning stiffness, and fatigue.

    Special tests include rheumatoid factor (RF) and anticitrullinated protein antibody (ACPA) testing, as well as joint imaging for erosions.
- *Osteoarthritis symptoms* include joint pain and stiffness, which increase with activity and improve with rest. Typically affects weight-bearing joints such as the knees and hips.

    Tests include X-rays that reveal joint space narrowing, osteophytes, and subchondral sclerosis.
- Signs and symptoms of *psoriatic arthritis* include joint discomfort and swelling, which may be asymmetrical. Associated with psoriatic skin lesions.

    Tests include clinical diagnosis based on imaging and the presence of skin lesions. A typical "Koebner phenomenon" which elicits a new psoriatic lesion formed by a controlled scratch in 10–20 days is also diagnostic of psoriasis.

COMPLICATIONS

- *Tophi*: Deposits of urate crystals that form lumps under the skin.
- *Kidney stones*: Caused by uric acid crystals in the kidneys.
- *Joint damage*: Chronic inflammation can lead to joint deformity and damage.

Proper management of hyperuricemia and gout involves a combination of medication, dietary modifications, and lifestyle changes to reduce symptoms and prevent complications.

CONCLUSION

Gout is a complex and multifaceted condition characterized by the accumulation of urate crystals in the joints, leading to intense pain, inflammation, and potential joint damage. As a form of inflammatory arthritis, gout's prevalence has risen in tandem with lifestyle changes, including dietary habits and increased life expectancy. Understanding the underlying pathophysiology, risk factors, and clinical presentation of gout is crucial for early diagnosis and effective management.

Throughout this chapter, we have explored the foundational aspects of gout, including genetic and environmental factors, epidemiology, and the biochemical mechanisms driving uric acid accumulation. We have also examined the clinical manifestations of gout, ranging from acute flares to chronic tophaceous gout, and the impact these have on patients' quality of life.

The introduction to gout sets the stage for a deeper exploration of its diagnostic criteria, treatment options, and preventive strategies, which are critical for improving patient outcomes. As we move forward, it is essential to keep in mind that gout is not only a medical condition but also a lifestyle-related disease, influenced by factors such as diet, alcohol consumption, and comorbidities like obesity and hypertension.

By fostering a comprehensive understanding of gout in its early stages, healthcare providers can better tailor interventions to manage the disease effectively, prevent complications, and enhance the overall well-being of those affected by this condition.

SUGGESTED READINGS

1. Chaudhary K, Malhotra K, Sowers J, Aroor A. Uric acid-key ingredient in the recipe for cardiorenal metabolic syndrome. Cardiorenal Med. 2013;3(3):208-20.
2. Maiuolo J, Oppedisano F, Gratteri S, Muscoli C, Mollace V. Regulation of uric acid metabolism and excretion. Int J Cardiol. 2016; 213:8-14.
3. Barr WG. Uric acid. Clinical Methods: In: Walker HK, Hall WD, Hurst JW (eds). The History, Physical, and Laboratory Examinations, 3rd edition. Boston: Butterworths; 1990.
4. Jin M, Yang F, Yang I, Yin Y, Luo JJ, Wang H, et al. Uric acid, hyperuricemia and vascular diseases. Front Biosci. 2012;17:656.
5. Su J, Wei Y, Liu M, Liu T, Li J, Ji Y, et al. Anti-hyperuricemic and nephroprotective effects of Rhizoma Dioscoreae septemlobae extracts and its main component dioscin via regulation of mOAT1, mURAT1 and mOCT2 in hypertensive mice. Arch Pharm Res. 2014; 37:1336-44.
6. Richette P, Doherty M, Pascual E, Barskova V, Becce F, Castañeda-Sanabria J, et al. 2016 updated EULAR evidence-based recommendations for the management of gout. Ann Rheum Dis. 2017; 76(1):29-42.
7. Riches PL, Wright AF, Ralston SH. Recent insights into the pathogenesis of hyperuricaemia and gout. Hum Mol Genet. 2009;18(R2): R177-84.
8. Doherty M. New insights into the epidemiology of gout. Rheumatology. 2009;48(suppl_2):ii2-8.
9. Feig DI, Kang DH, Johnson RJ. Uric acid and cardiovascular risk. N Engl J Med. 2008;359(17):1811-21.
10. Annemans L, Spaepen E, Gaskin M, Bonnemaire M, Malier V, Gilbert T, et al. Gout in the UK and Germany: Prevalence, comorbidities and management in general practice 2000–2005. Ann Rheum Dis. 2008;67(7):960-6.
11. Leow MK. Uric acid and cardiovascular risk. N Engl J Med. 2009;360(5):538-9.
12. Choi HK, Mount DB, Reginato AM. Pathogenesis of gout. Ann Intern Med. 2005;143(7):499-516.
13. Estiverne C, Mandal AK, Mount DB. Molecular pathophysiology of uric acid homeostasis. Semin Nephrol. 2020;40(6):535-49.

14. Zhu Y, Pandya BJ, Choi HK. Prevalence of gout and hyperuricemia in the US general population: The National Health and Nutrition Examination Survey 2007–2008. Arthritis Rheum. 2011;63(10): 3136-41.
15. Kundu AK. Gout in Indian Scenario. Med Update. 2013;23:445-58.
16. Chopra A, Patil J, Billempelly V, Relwani J, Tandle HS. Prevalence of rheumatic diseases in a rural population in western India: A WHO-ILAR COPCORD Study. J Assoc Physicians India. 2001;49: 240-6.
17. Matthew A, Danda D. Clinical profile of young onset gout in India. Vellore experience. J Ind Rheum Assoc. 2004:12-8.
18. de Oliveira EP, Burini RC. High plasma uric acid concentration: causes and consequences. Diabetol Metab Syndr. 2012;4(1):1-7.
19. Cuppari L. Guia de Nutrição: Nutrição Clínica do Adulto. Português: Manole. 2005. p. 474.
20. Choi HK, Atkinson K, Karlson EW, Willett W, Curhan G. Purine-rich foods, dairy and protein intake, and the risk of gout in men. N Engl J Med. 2004;350(11):1093-103.
21. Johnson RJ, Rideout BA. Uric acid and diet—insights into the epidemic of cardiovascular disease. N Engl J Med. 2004;350(11): 1071-3.
22. Saag KG, Choi H. Epidemiology, risk factors, and lifestyle modifications for gout. Arthritis Res Ther. 2006;8(1):1-7.
23. Choi HK, Curhan G. Beer, liquor, and wine consumption and serum uric acid level: The Third National Health and Nutrition Examination Survey. Arthritis Care Res (Hoboken). 2004;51(6):1023-9.
24. Drum DE, Goldman PA, Jankowski CB. Elevation of serum uric acid as a clue to alcohol abuse. Arch Intern Med. 1981;141(4):477-9.
25. Sharpe CR. A case-control study of alcohol consumption and drinking behaviour in patients with acute gout. CMAJ. 1984;131(6):563.
26. Vandenberg MK, Moxley G, Breitbach SA, Roberts WN. Gout attacks in chronic alcoholics occur at lower serum urate levels than in nonalcoholics. J Rheumatol. 1994;21(4):700-4.
27. Eastmond CJ, Garton M, Robins S, Riddoch S. The effects of alcoholic beverages on urate metabolism in gout sufferers. Rheumatology. 1995;34(8):756-9.
28. Faller J, Fox IH. Ethanol-induced hyperuricemia: evidence for increased urate production by activation of adenine nucleotide turnover. N Engl J Med. 1982;307(26):1598-602.

29. Puig JG, Fox IH. Ethanol-induced activation of adenine nucleotide turnover. Evidence for a role of acetate. J Clin Invest. 1984;74(3):936-41.
30. Hanna BE, Hamed JM, Touhala LM. Serum uric Acid in smokers. Oman Med J. 2008;23(4):269.
31. Haj Mouhamed D, Ezzaher A, Neffati F, Douki W, Gaha L, Najjar MF. Effect of cigarette smoking on plasma uric acid concentrations. Environ Health Prev Med. 2011;16:307-12.
32. Tomita M, Mizuno S, Yokota K. Increased levels of serum uric acid among ex-smokers. J Epidemiol. 2008;18(3):132-4.
33. Raja S, Kumar A, Aahooja RD, Thakuria U, Ochani S, Shaukat F. Frequency of hyperuricemia and its risk factors in the adult population. Cureus. 2019;11(3):e4198.
34. Park DY, Kim YS, Ryu SH, Jin YS. The association between sedentary behavior, physical activity and hyperuricemia. Vasc Health Risk Manag. 2019;15:291-9.
35. Ben Salem C, Slim R, Fathallah N, Hmouda H. Drug-induced hyperuricaemia and gout. Rheumatology. 2017;56(5):679-88.

CHAPTER **2**

Metabolism of Uric Acid

Nindiya Kapoor Mehra, Shivam Mehra, Sumedha Shinde, Sachiti Sachin Kale

INTRODUCTION

Uric acid is a vital metabolite in humans and other animals, primarily as the end product of purine metabolism. Understanding the metabolism of uric acid is crucial, as imbalances in its production or excretion can lead to various health issues, including gout, kidney stones, and other metabolic disorders.

Interestingly, while many animals have an enzyme called uricase that further breaks down uric acid into allantoin, humans and some other primates lack this enzyme due to evolutionary mutations. This absence makes humans more prone to uric acid-related disorders but also provides certain antioxidant benefits.

OVERVIEW OF URIC ACID METABOLISM IN THE HUMAN BODY

In the human body, uric acid metabolism is a complex process involving the breakdown of purines, which are found in many foods and also occur naturally in the body. Here is a detailed overview of how this process works.

Purine Breakdown

- *Source of purines*: Purines are obtained from the diet (e.g., meat, fish, and certain vegetables) and are also synthesized in the body.
- *Catabolism*: Purines are broken down through a series of enzymatic reactions. The key enzyme involved that catalyzes the conversion of hypoxanthine to xanthine and subsequently xanthine to uric acid is xanthine oxidase.

Formation of Uric Acid

- *Xanthine from hypoxanthine*: Xanthine oxidase enzyme converts hypoxanthine to xanthine.
- *Uric acid from xanthine*: Xanthine oxidase oxidizes Xanthine to form uric acid.

Excretion of Uric Acid

- *Bloodstream*: Once formed, uric acid is released into the bloodstream.
- *Kidneys*: The kidneys filter the blood, reabsorbing some uric acid and excreting the rest in the urine. Approximately 67% of uric acid is excreted through the kidneys.
- *Intestines*: The remaining 33% of uric acid gets excreted through the intestines, where it is broken down by bacteria.

Regulation of Uric Acid Levels

- *Balance*: Normally, there is a balance between uric acid production and excretion, maintaining healthy levels in the blood.
- *Hyperuricemia*: Hyperuricemia, that is, raised levels of uric acid in the blood can occur due to overproduction or underexcretion. This condition can lead to gout, characterized by the precipitation of urate crystals in tissues and joints, causing pain and inflammation.

- *Hypouricemia*: Hypouricemia, that is, smaller levels of uric acid in the blood are less common and can be due to certain medical conditions or genetic factors.

STEPS IN URIC ACID METABOLISM

Purine Breakdown and Formation of Uric Acid: Endogenous Purine Metabolism

- *Adenine metabolism pathway*:
  - *Adenine nucleotide breakdown*: A component of adenosine monophosphate (AMP), adenosine diphosphate (ADP), and adenosine triphosphate (ATP) is adenine. AMP is dephosphorylated to adenosine by the enzyme 5′-nucleotidase. Inosine is then formed by the deamination of adenosine by the enzyme adenosine deaminase.
  - *Inosine conversion*: Inosine is hydrolyzed to hypoxanthine and ribose by the enzyme purine nucleoside phosphorylase (PNP).
  - *Hypoxanthine metabolism*: Xanthine oxidase converts hypoxanthine to xanthine. Xanthine oxidase further oxidizes xanthine to uric acid **(Figs. 1A and B)**.
- *Guanine metabolism pathway*:
  - *Guanine nucleotide breakdown*: Guanosine monophosphate (GMP), guanosine diphosphate (GDP), and guanosine triphosphate (GTP) all contain guanine as a component. GMP is dephosphorylated to guanosine by the enzyme 5′-nucleotidase. Guanosine is hydrolyzed to guanine and ribose by the enzyme PNP.
  - *Guanine conversion*: Guanine deaminase (guanase) enzyme is responsible for the deamination of guanine to xanthine.
  - *Xanthine metabolism*: Postconversion of guanine to xanthine, xanthine oxidase enzyme oxidizes xanthine to form uric acid **(Figs. 1A and B)**.

CHAPTER 2: Metabolism of Uric Acid

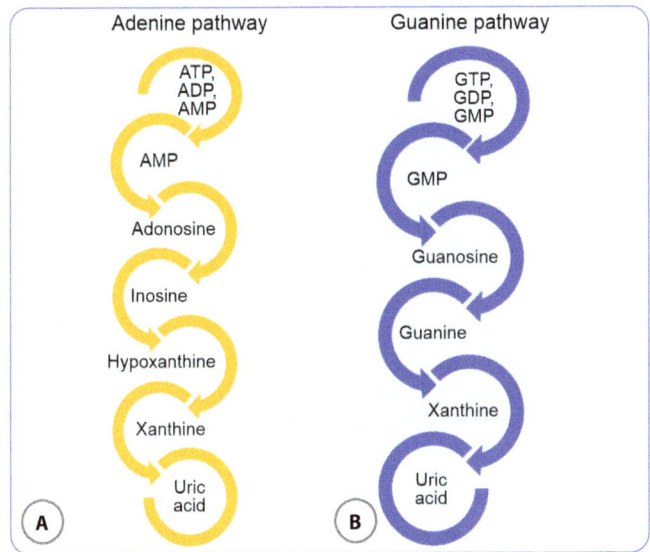

Figs. 1A and B: The adenine and guanine pathway of uric acid formation.

In normal human physiological conditions, uric acid exists as urate. The normal range of uric acid in males is 2.5–7.0 mg/dL and in females is 1.5–6.0 mg/dL, respectively. Further, the renal excretion of urate (almost 200–300 mg/day) happens as it is easily transformed to allantoic acid and ammonia.

The metabolism of adenine and guanine follows distinct but converging pathways that ultimately lead to the formation of uric acid. Both pathways involve dephosphorylation, deamination, and oxidation steps, with key enzymes such as purine deaminase, PNP, and xanthine oxidase playing crucial roles in the process.

Excretion of Uric Acid

Uric acid excretion is a critical component of its metabolism, ensuring that uric acid levels in the body remain balanced and

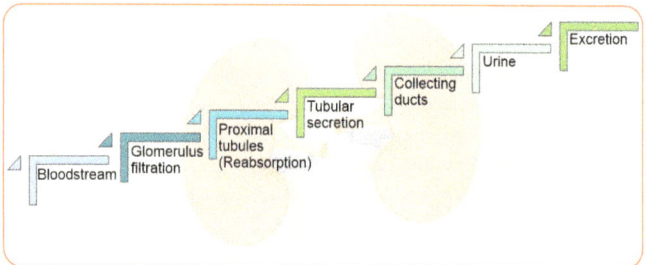

Fig. 2: Schematic representation of uric acid excretion through kidneys.

preventing the accumulation that can lead to conditions like gout **(Fig. 2)**. Here is a detailed overview of how uric acid is excreted:

- *Filtration and reabsorption in the kidneys*:
  - *Glomerular filtration*:
    - Uric acid is filtered out of the blood through the glomeruli, which are tiny blood vessels in the kidneys.
    - Approximately 100% of uric acid is filtered from the blood at this stage.
  - *Reabsorption*:
    - After filtration, in the proximal tubules of the kidneys, a significant portion of the uric acid is reabsorbed back into the bloodstream.
    - Specific transport proteins such as urate transporter 1 (URAT1) and glucose transporter 9 (GLUT9) mediate this reabsorption process.
  - *Secretion in the kidneys*: Tubular secretion—
    - A portion of the reabsorbed uric acid is secreted back into the tubular fluid to be excreted in the urine.
    - This secretion involves various renal transporters, including organic anion transporter 1 (OAT1) and OAT3.

- *Final excretion:* Urine—
  - Ultimately, in the urine, about 10% of the filtered uric acid gets excreted.
  - This process ensures that excess uric acid is removed from the body, helping to maintain proper uric acid levels in the blood.
- *Intestinal excretion*: Bacterial breakdown—
  - The remaining uric acid that is not expelled by the kidneys is transported to the intestines.
  - In the intestines, uric acid is broken down by bacteria and excreted in the feces.

Uric acid excretion involves a balance of filtration, reabsorption, and secretion processes in the kidneys, with additional breakdown and excretion in the intestines. Efficient excretion is crucial for maintaining healthy uric acid levels and preventing disorders such as gout and kidney stones. Factors such as diet, hydration, genetics, medications, and health conditions can influence the excretion process.

HYPERURICEMIA AND METABOLIC DISORDERS

Purine metabolism leads to the formation of uric acid. Due to the absence in the activity of uricase enzyme in humans, serum uric acid (SUA) levels tend to increase as compared to other mammals. Due to elevated SUA, it relates and predicts development of gout and renal calculi, cardiovascular diseases, obesity, and hypertension.

Uric acid excretion happens mainly through the kidneys and the leftover through the intestines. The disparity in the formation and elimination of uric acid results in the metabolic disorders mentioned above.

Many studies have shown that uric acid plays an important role in scavenging reactive oxygen species (ROS) and is a major antioxidant in humans. However, multiple diseases being linked to elevated uric acid levels have also been in the picture.

Thus, the oxidant-antioxidant paradox in case of uric acid has been a long-standing debate.

One way to explain this paradox could be that a shoot up in uric acid levels can be regarded as an attempted protective response by the host, but some literature points to the fact that uric acid may function either as an antioxidant (primarily in plasma) or pro-oxidant (primarily within the cell).

The concentration of uric acid depends on uric acid metabolism in terms of these four aspects—(1) purine intake in the diet, (2) endogenous purine metabolism, (3) urate excretion through kidneys, and (4) urate excretion through the intestine. Of these, the major mutable risk factor is diet intake that determines SUA concentration. Purine-rich foods include seafood, organ meats, beer, and other meats. In particular, fructose rich foods in the diet may also lead to hyperuricemia.

Phosphorylation of fructose to fructose 1-phosphate increases the AMP pool at the cost of ATP. The AMP then increases uric acid by entering the purine metabolic pathway **(Flowchart 1)**. Fructokinase catalyzes phosphorylation of fructose, and is different from other hexokinases as it does not get inhibited by the product. As a consequence, fructose consumption leads to fast exhaustion of ATP and heightened formation of uric acid in the liver.

Added sugars consumption in India has increased considerably in the past decades which is in sync with the increase in metabolic disorders. Added sugars, mainly fructose-containing sugars, have had damaging impact on diseases such as gout, type 2 diabetes, and cardiovascular disease. Other modifiers that can increase SUA are vitamin C, caffeine, and alcohol. Alcohol (ethanol) is known to increase SUA and decrease uric acid excretion. High-dose vitamin C reduces SUA levels by having a uricosuric effect. Caffeine decreases SUA concentration by inhibiting xanthine oxidase activity **(Flowchart 1)**.

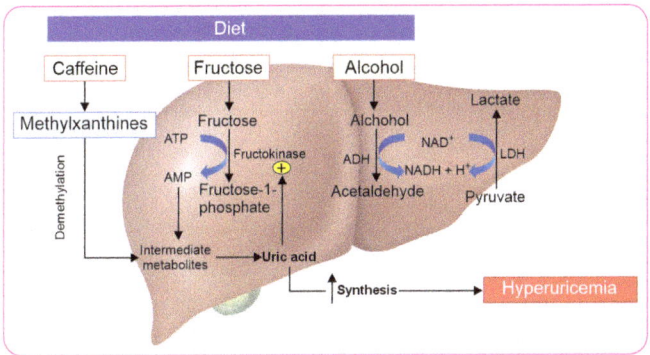

Flowchart 1: The endogenous production of uric acid and hyperuricemia through metabolism of caffeine, fructose, and alcohol.

(ADH: alcohol dehydrogenase; AMP: adenosine monophosphate; ATP: adenosine triphosphate; LDH: lactate dehydrogenase; NAD: nicotinamide adenine dinucleotide)

COMPARISON OF NORMAL URIC ACID METABOLISM VERSUS HYPERURICEMIA METABOLISM

Here is a comparison between normal uric acid metabolism and hyperuricemia metabolism (**Flowcharts 2 and 3**).

Normal Uric Acid Metabolism

- *Purine intake and synthesis*: Purines come from dietary sources (meat, fish, vegetables) and are also synthesized by the body.
- *Purine breakdown*:
  - Purines are broken down into hypoxanthine.
  - Xanthine oxidase converts hypoxanthine to xanthine.
  - Xanthine oxidase converts xanthine to uric acid.

CHAPTER 2: Metabolism of Uric Acid

```
Dietary purines              Endogenous purines
      ↓                              ↓
   Breakdown                      Breakdown
      ↓                              ↓
  Hypoxanthine                  Hypoxanthine
      ↓                              ↓
    Xanthine                       Xanthine
      ↓                              ↓
    Uric acid                      Uric acid
      ↓                              ↓
   Bloodstream                   Bloodstream
      ↓                              ↓
    Kidneys                        Kidneys
      ↓                              ↓
Filter and excrete (Urine)   Filter and excrete (Urine)
      ↓                              ↓
 Intestinal excretion          Intestinal excretion

   Balance maintained           Balance maintained
```

Flowchart 2: Normal uric acid metabolism.

```
   Dietary purines              Endogenous purines
  (Excessive intake)            (Increased synthesis)
         ↓                              ↓
     Breakdown                       Breakdown
         ↓                              ↓
   Hypoxanthine                    Hypoxanthine
   (Overproduction)                (Overproduction)
         ↓                              ↓
   Xanthine (Increased            Xanthine (Increased
activity of xanthine oxidase)  activity of xanthine oxidase)
         ↓                              ↓
  Uric acid (Elevated levels)   Uric acid (Elevated levels)
         ↓                              ↓
 Bloodstream (Elevated levels) Bloodstream (Elevated levels)
         ↓                              ↓
  Kidneys (Reduced excretion)   Kidneys (Reduced excretion)
         ↓                              ↓
   Reduced filtering (Urine)     Reduced filtering (Urine)
         ↓                              ↓
    Intestinal excretion           Intestinal excretion

  Hyperuricemia—Gout risk       Hyperuricemia—Tophi risk
```

Flowchart 3: Hyperuricemia metabolism.

- *Uric acid excretion*:
  - Uric acid enters the bloodstream.
  - The kidneys filter the blood, reabsorbing some uric acid and excreting the rest in the urine (about two-thirds).
  - Excretion of leftover uric acid happens through the intestines (about one-third).

Hyperuricemia Metabolism

- *Purine intake and synthesis*:
  - Excessive purine intake from diet.
  - Increased synthesis due to genetic factors or cell turnover.
- *Purine breakdown*:
  - Overproduction of hypoxanthine and xanthine
  - Heightened activity of xanthine oxidase causes higher levels of uric acid.
- *Uric acid excretion*:
  - Impaired kidney function or medications reduce uric acid excretion.
  - Genetic mutations affect renal transport proteins, decreasing uric acid excretion.
- *Resulting hyperuricemia*:
  - Elevated uric acid levels in the blood
  - Formation of monosodium urate crystals
  - Deposition in joints and tissues causing gout and tophi

CONCLUSION

The metabolism of uric acid is a critical biological process that plays a significant role in human health, particularly in the context of disorders such as gout and hyperuricemia. This chapter has provided an in-depth exploration of how uric acid is produced, transported, and excreted in the body, as well as the factors that can disrupt its balance.

We have examined the key pathways involved in the synthesis of uric acid, emphasizing the role of purine metabolism and the enzyme xanthine oxidase in converting hypoxanthine to xanthine and subsequently to uric acid. Additionally, we have discussed how uric acid is primarily excreted through the kidneys, with a smaller portion eliminated through the intestines, highlighting the significance of renal function in maintaining uric acid homeostasis.

As we conclude this chapter, it is evident that the metabolism of uric acid is a complex process influenced by multiple biological and environmental factors. A thorough understanding of these processes is essential for clinicians and researchers to design better therapeutic approaches to manage and prevent uric acid-related disorders. As we move forward, further research into the regulation of uric acid metabolism and its broader implications in human health will be vital in advancing our knowledge and improving patient care.

SUGGESTED READINGS

1. Stone TW, Simmonds A. Purines: Basic and clinical aspects. Germany: Springer Science & Business Media; 2012.
2. Newcombe DS. Gout: Basic science and clinical practice. Germany: Springer Science & Business Media; 2012.
3. Fathallah-Shaykh SA, Cramer MT. Uric acid and the kidney. Pediatr Nephrol. 2014;29(6):999-1008.
4. El Din UA, Salem MM, Abdulazim DO. Uric acid in the pathogenesis of metabolic, renal, and cardiovascular diseases: A review. J Adv Res. 2017;8(5):537-48.
5. Katsiki N, Dimitriadis GD, Mikhailidis DP. Serum uric acid and diabetes: from pathophysiology to cardiovascular disease. Curr Pharm Design. 2021;27(16):1941-51.
6. Mitra SP. The biochemical & physiological implication of gout. Am J Biopharmacol Biochem Life Sci. 2012;1:1-35.

CHAPTER 3

Indian Communities and their Effect on Elevated Uric Acid Levels: A Multicentric Study

Sachin Yaswant Kale, Kamal Mehra, Shivam Mehra, Nindiya Kapoor Mehra, Bharat Veer Manchanda

INTRODUCTION

This book is one of the first attempts to provide estimates on the prevalence of high levels of serum uric acid in different religious Indian communities namely Hindu, Sikh, Christian, and Muslim, a prerequisite for knowing the risk of development of gout amongst them with a multicentric approach.

DETAILS OF THE STUDY SAMPLE

The study covered in this chapter was conducted during the period from April 2018 to May 2021, the subjects enrolled in this study were divided into four groups (group I, group II, group III and group IV). Informed consent was obtained from all individual participants included in the study. In accordance with the Helsinki Declaration of 1975 (as revised in 2013) and the ethical standards of the responsible committee on human experimentation (institutional and national), all the procedures were followed. A total of 10,337 patients were part of this study. All patients' blood samples were collected after informed consent following strict aseptic protocol and processed in a certified standardized clinical biochemical laboratory.

Group I was the Hindu community composed of 8,313 volunteers, their mean age being 45 years. Group II was the Sikh community composed of 362 volunteers, their mean age being 46 years. Group III was the Christian community composed of 571 volunteers, the mean age of the group being 52 years. Group IV was the Muslim community composed of 1,091 volunteers, the mean age of the group being 42 years **(Table 1 and Figs. 1 and 2)**.

This study recorded the complete history of patients, including name, age, religion, gender **(Table 2 and Fig. 3)**, vegetarian or nonvegetarian **(Table 3 and Fig. 4)**, consumption of alcohol, smoker or nonsmoker, type of lifestyle

Table 1: Data disposition for religion (all data).		
	Numbers	Percentage (%)
Christian	571	5.5
Hindu	8,313	80.4
Islam	1,091	10.6
Sikh	362	3.5
Total	**10,337**	

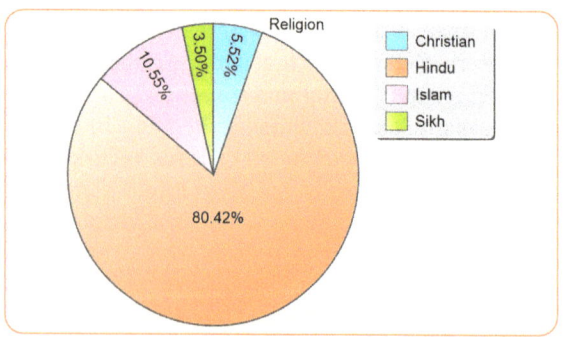

Fig. 1: Religion of the study sample (%, n = 10,337).

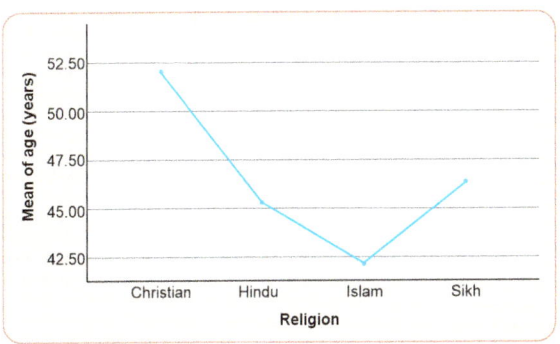

Fig. 2: Mean age of the study sample in different religions (%, $n = 10,337$).

Table 2: Gender of study sample ($n = 10,337$).

	Numbers	Percentage (%)
Male	5,986	57.9
Female	4,351	42.1
Total	**10,337**	

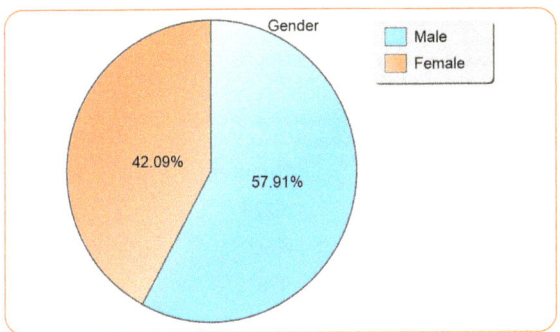

Fig. 3: Gender of the study sample (%, $n = 10,337$).

(Table 4 and Fig. 5), any comorbidities, previous history of gout, any joint pain, and drug allergies.

Data Disposition

Analysis dataset includes 10,337 study samples.

Table 3: Dietary habits of study sample (n = 10,337).

	Numbers	Percentage (%)
Vegetarian	5,474	53.0
Non-vegetarian	4,863	47.0
Total	**10,337**	

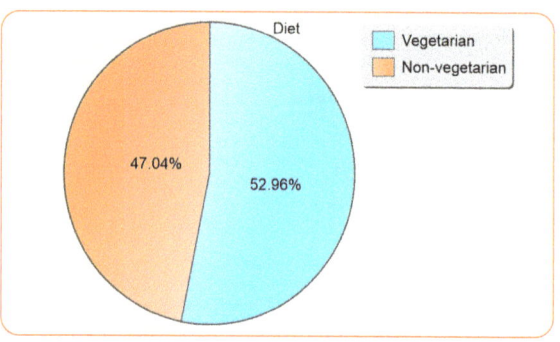

Fig. 4: Dietary habits of the study sample (%, n = 10,337).

Table 4: Lifestyle of study sample (n = 10,337).

	Numbers	Percentage (%)
Light physical activity	3,229	31.2
Moderate physical activity	4,669	45.2
Vigorous physical activity	976	9.4
Sedentary	1,463	14.2
Total	**10,337**	

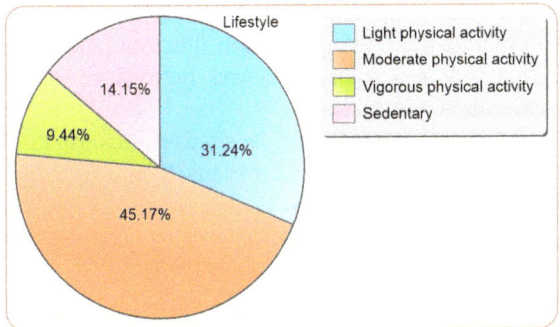

Fig. 5: Lifestyle of the study sample (%, $n = 10{,}337$).

Demography of Analysis Dataset

For colorimetric measurement of uric acid, fasting blood and random urine samples were obtained from all four groups.

Inclusion and Exclusion Criteria

Inclusion criteria included all the hospital inpatient and outpatient departments (IPD and OPD) patients who were willing to participate in the study and above 18 years of age.

The exclusion criteria of this study included age < 20 years and >65 years having deranged laboratory values, gout, pregnancy, stroke, kidney diseases, severe degenerative diseases, cancer, mental deficiency, and bedridden patients. Also, we excluded patients who were not willing to participate in the study.

RESULTS OF THE MULTICENTRIC STUDY

Standard statistical methods were used to evaluate the results. These included mean, range (minimum-maximum), standard deviation (SD), linear regression analysis using Pearson correlation coefficient r, and Student's t-test with computer software programs including Microsoft Excel 2003 and SPSS 11.5 to evaluate the relation between different parameters of both groups. At $p > 0.05$, differences between observations were considered nonsignificant.

The mean serum uric acid levels were highest in Sikhs (6.5 mg%, n = 662) followed by Christians (6.18 mg%, n = 1,071) Hindus (5.65 mg%, n = 16,313), and Muslims (5.55 mg%, n = 2,091) **(Fig. 6)**. Lifestyle, diet, drinking, and smoking habits had a role to play in the levels of uric acid as found out in our study. 100% Muslims consumed a nonvegetarian diet followed by 89.5% Christians. Heavy drinking was highest in Sikhs at around 10.2%. Further, 15.7% Hindus were current smokers followed by 13.8% Sikhs who smoked at present. The percentage of Hindus was highest in sedentary lifestyle (15.4%).

Hyperuricemia and gout are pressing health issues despite effective therapies available. Although the condition is influenced by genetic factors, many reports suggest that external factors such as alcohol consumption, smoking habits, nonvegetarian diet, and lifestyle also play a role in modulating gout. In our report, we seek to study the prevalence of uric acid

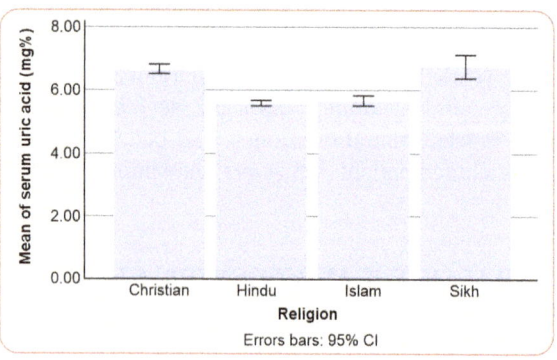

Fig. 6: Mean serum uric acid of the study sample in different religions (%, n = 10,337).

levels amongst different religious Indian communities. This is the first report linking communities and their lifestyle habits to uric acid levels. The highest uric acid levels were reported in Sikhs which was influenced by more consumption of fish and meat, higher percentage of binge drinking, sedentary lifestyle, and higher percentage of joint disorders. This was followed by Christians, Hindus, and Muslims. Our study is a unique study that links religious communities and their lifestyle habits to uric acid levels and hence, their predisposition toward gout.

DISCUSSION

In India, studies on gout in different communities and populations are lacking. As there is less data, we do not have much clarity on how different Indian patients with gout behave in response to different drugs. On one hand, many physicians and doctors are not adequately trained to manage gout properly, while on the other hand patients take nonsteroidal anti-inflammatory drugs (NSAIDs) on their own. There is a need for such community-based, region-based, and gender-based studies that can guide rheumatologists and physicians toward prescribing the right treatment to the patient.

For example, findings of a study performed in Kerala showed that gout had a definite male prevalence. It was observed that initially gout manifested in a single joint, mainly the ankle joint. But in totality, the first metatarsophalangeal joint was the most common joint to be affected. Approximately > 90% of the study population had this joint affected at some point of the disease. The study also concluded that many patients secreted low uric acid levels but had higher occurrence of renal calculi.

Other examples of variation in prevalence of gout with geographic differences are the results of the Community Oriented Program for the Control of Rheumatic Diseases

(COPCORD). These studies reported a very low prevalence of gout in Jammu, India, that is, 0.19%. A lower incidence rate of gout was reported in a rural population in village Bhigwan, Pune in Western India. Gout was diagnosed in 0.12% in the studied population, and the study reported not a single case of gout in women.

Thus, it is very crucial to have studies such as community-based studies, geography-based studies, religion-based studies to identify patients of gout and prescribe them with the right kind of treatment.

CONCLUSION

Overall, our study of 10,337 patients demonstrated that the serum uric acid levels varied from one Indian community to another due to varying external factors like diet, age, lifestyle, and addictions. Thus, lifestyle modification in communities with higher serum uric acid levels is highly advocated and this may reduce the healthcare burden of gouty arthritis in these communities.

SUGGESTED READINGS

1. Paul BJ, Rahman TM, Sudheesh T. Clinical study of gout in North Kerala. Indian J Rheumatol. 2009;4(4):149-52.
2. Mahajan A, Jasrotia DS, Manhas AS, Jamwal SS. (2003). Prevalence of major rheumatic disorders in Jammu. [online] Available from https://www.jkscience.org/archive/Volume52/Prevalence%20of%20Major%20Rheumatic%20Disorders%20in%20jammu.pdf [Last accessed August, 2024].
3. Chopra A, Patil J, Billempelly V, Relwani J, Tandle HS. Prevalence of rheumatic diseases in a rural population in western India: a WHO-ILAR COPCORD Study. J Assoc Physicians India. 2001;49:240-6.

CHAPTER 4

Increase in Incidence of Uric Acid Levels and Gout Postmenopause

Kamal Mehra, Nindiya Kapoor Mehra, Shivam Mehra, Smruti Sachin Kale

INTRODUCTION

Gout, a form of inflammatory arthritis, is traditionally associated with men, but it increasingly affects women, particularly after menopause. The interplay between hormonal changes during menopause and the onset or exacerbation of gout is an emerging area of interest in medical research and clinical practice. Understanding this relationship is essential for developing effective prevention and treatment strategies for postmenopausal women.

RELATIONSHIP BETWEEN GOUT AND MENOPAUSE

Menopause can be described as a progressive change from pre- to postmenopause with modifications in the levels of estrogen and progesterone that not only takes a toll on a woman's health by impacting cardiovascular function, osteoporosis, and sexual dysfunction but also affects the SUA levels. Multiple studies have independently shown the effect

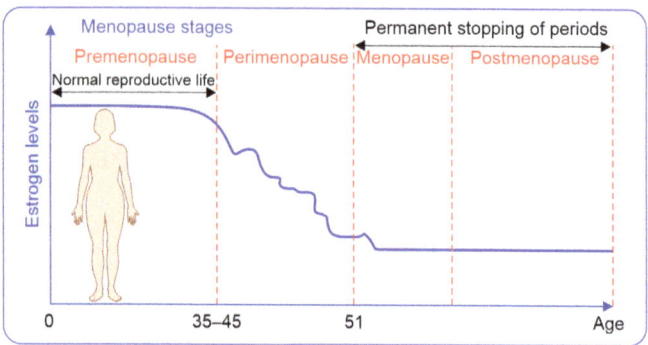

Fig. 1: Estrogen levels and stages of menopause.

of estrogen depletion postmenopause has an impact on the excretion of uric acid through the kidneys. The Third National Health and Nutrition Examination Survey conducted from 1988 to 1994 presented data that demonstrated that menopause was associated with hyperuricemia. The levels of serum uric acid were higher in women postmenopause as compared to women premenopause, a data of 7,662 US women (aged 20 years and above) by 0.34–0.36 mg/dL. Further, this study also demonstrated that use of postmenopausal hormone reduced uric acid levels in women after menopause.

Studies in Indian postmenopausal women have also been conducted and they indicate the same results. A study done on 150 postmenopausal Indian women showed that these women had more joint diseases with around 1.3% of these women having gout **(Fig. 1)**.

IMPACT OF MENOPAUSE ON METABOLISM OF URIC ACID

Uric acid metabolism in menopausal women involves several steps, including its production, excretion, and the influence of

hormonal changes, particularly the decline in estrogen. Here is a detailed explanation:
- *Estrogen and uric acid excretion*: Estrogen facilitates uric acid excretion by enhancing its renal clearance. This process involves:
  - *Increased glomerular filtration*: Estrogen increases the glomerular filtration rate (GFR), leading to more uric acid being filtered out of the blood.
  - *Reduced reabsorption*: Estrogen reduces uric acid reabsorption in the renal tubules, allowing more uric acid to be excreted in the urine.
- *Postmenopausal decline in estrogen*: After menopause, the decline in estrogen levels leads to:
  - *Decreased GFR*: The reduction in estrogen causes a decrease in GFR, resulting in less uric acid being filtered out of the blood.
  - *Increased reabsorption*: Reabsorption of uric acid in the renal tubules takes place due to low estrogen levels, causing elevated levels of uric acid in the serum **(Flowchart 1)**.

In menopausal women, the metabolism of uric acid is influenced by a decline in estrogen, leading to decreased excretion of uric acid by the kidneys and heightened levels of uric acid in the serum. This process is further affected by factors such as weight gain, comorbid conditions, and certain medications, increasing the risk of hyperuricemia and gout.

RISK FACTORS FOR HYPERURICEMIA AND GOUT IN POSTMENOPAUSAL WOMEN

There are multiple factors that could be considered responsible for gout in postmenopausal women.

Some of these factors include:
- *Hormonal changes*: Estrogen is known to have a uricosuric effect, meaning it helps in the renal excretion of uric acid.

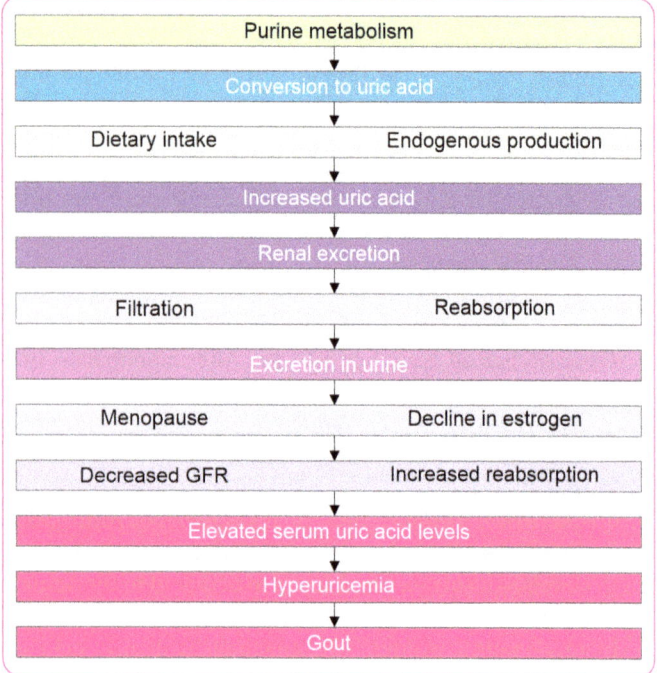

Flowchart 1: The uric acid metabolism in menopausal women.

Postmenopause, estrogen levels drop, leading to decreased uric acid excretion and consequently higher uric acid levels in the blood.
- *Decreased renal function*: There has been an association between aging and a reduction in kidney function. Postmenopausal women might experience a further decrease in renal function, which can impair the kidneys' ability to excrete uric acid efficiently.
- *Weight gain*: Menopause is often accompanied by weight gain, particularly an increase in visceral fat. This can lead to insulin resistance, which is associated with elevated levels

of uric acid. Obesity itself is a risk factor for hyperuricemia and gout (high levels of uric acid).
- *Dietary changes*: Changes in dietary habits postmenopause, such as increased consumption of purine-rich foods (e.g., seafood, red meat) and fructose (found in processed foods and sugary drinks), can contribute to elevated uric acid levels.
- *Decreased physical activity*: A decrease in physical activity, which is common postmenopause, can lead to weight gain and metabolic changes that increase uric acid levels.
- *Metabolic syndrome*: Postmenopausal women are at an increased risk for metabolic syndrome, a bunch of conditions that include insulin resistance, abdominal obesity, hypertension, and abnormal levels of lipids in the bloodstream. Metabolic syndrome is strongly associated with elevated uric acid levels.
- *Medications*: Certain medications that are more commonly used postmenopause, such as diuretics, can cause an increase in the levels of uric acid. The mechanism of action of diuretics is that they reduce blood volume by increasing urine output, but they also decrease the excretion of uric acid.
- *Genetic factors*: Genetic predisposition can play a role in uric acid levels. Some women may have a genetic makeup that predisposes them to higher uric acid levels, and this can become more pronounced postmenopause.

MANAGEMENT AND PREVENTION OF HYPERURICEMIA AND GOUT IN POSTMENOPAUSAL WOMEN

- *Dietary modifications*:
  - *Reduce purine intake*: Decreasing consumption of foods that are high in purines, such as seafood, red meat, and alcohol, mainly beer.

- *Increase intake of low-fat dairy*: Intake of dairy products which are low fat can help reduce the levels of uric acid.
    - *Hydration*: Drinking plenty of water to help the renal excretion of uric acid.
- *Medications*:
    - *Uric acid-lowering drugs*: Allopurinol, febuxostat, or probenecid is uric acid lowering medications that may be prescribed.
    - *Anti-inflammatory drugs*: Nonsteroidal anti-inflammatory drugs (NSAIDs), colchicine, or corticosteroids may be used during acute gout attacks to lessen inflammation and pain.
- *Lifestyle changes*:
    - *Weight management*: Healthy weight maintenance through diet and exercise
    - *Regular physical activity*: Performing physical activity regularly to boost overall health and reduce the risk of gout.
- *Monitoring and regular check-ups*:
    - *Uric acid levels*: Consistent monitoring of levels of uric acid to manage and adjust treatment as needed.
    - *Kidney function*: Monitoring kidney function to ensure effective excretion of uric acid.
- *Managing comorbid conditions*:
    - Proper management of conditions like hypertension, diabetes, and hyperlipidemia, which can impact uric acid levels and gout risk **(Figs. 2A and B)**.

RESEARCH STUDIES ON URIC ACID AND MENOPAUSE

A Study of Nonobese Healthy Women with Menopause

In this study, 50 women before menopause and 88 women postmenopause were evaluated for serum uric levels. These

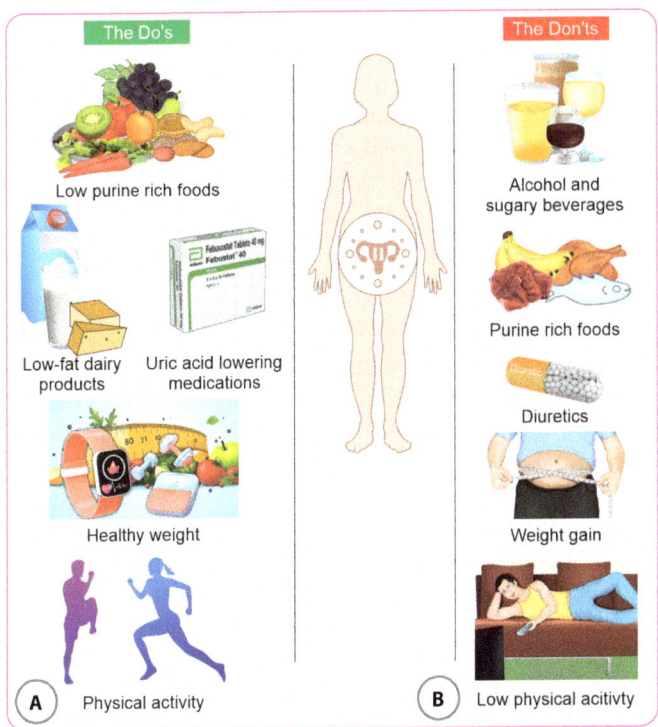

Figs. 2A and B: The Do's and Don'ts for the prevention and management of hyperuricemia in postmenopausal women.

women were white women, nonobese who went through a glucose tolerance test intravenously. The concentration of uric acid was significantly higher in postmenopausal as compared to premenopausal women. The data was adjusted for variable factors such as age and body mass index (BMI). After adjusting, it showed a highly significant independent difference between the groups. Also, this study showed that BMI was an important forecaster of serum uric acid levels in premenopausal women. Postmenopausal women were found to be more insulin-resistant, and there was a reasonable association between uric acid and insulin resistance syndrome in both the groups. The study concluded that increases in serum uric acid in postmenopausal women may result from changes in metabolism as a consequence of the menopause, and may be associated with the increased risk of coronary heart disease (CHD) seen in these women.

A Study Conducted to Understand the Association of Serum Uric Acid and Bone Mineral Density in Postmenopausal Women

In this study, data from 328 postmenopausal women (mean age, 57.3 ± 6.5 years; mean serum uric acid level, 4.6 ± 1.0 mg/dL) was collected. The participants were divided into three groups based on levels of serum uric acid. Results—blood urea nitrogen, serum creatinine, and serum triglyceride levels were significantly higher in the upper tertiles of uric acid levels. A cross-sectional analysis showed no significant correlation between the serum uric acid levels and BMD in the spine and femoral neck. Longitudinal analysis of data from 186 women with follow-up examinations at a mean interval of 14.6 months also revealed no difference in reduction in both spine and femoral neck BMD between tertile groups of serum uric acid.

A Prospective Study to Understand the Relation between Menopause, Postmenopausal Hormone Use and Risk of Gout

In the Nurses' Health Study, the association between menopause, age at menopause, postmenopausal hormone use, and risk of self-reported physician-diagnosed incident gout among 92,535 women without gout at baseline was examined.
- *Results*: During 16 years of follow-up, 1,703 incident gout cases were recorded. The incidence rate of gout increased

from 0.6 per 1,000 person-years in women < 45 years of age to 2.5 in women ≥ 75 years of age (p for trend < 0.001). Compared with premenopausal women, postmenopausal women had a higher risk of the occurrence of gout. Hormone use in postmenopausal women had a decreased risk of gout.
- *Conclusion*: These findings point out that the risk of gout increases due to menopause, whereas use of hormone therapy after menopause modestly reduces gout risk.

A Study Showing Elevated Levels of Uric Acid in Postmenopausal Women Associated with Inflammation and Other Adverse Outcomes

This study was performed to understand the association between serum uric acid levels, markers of inflammation and coronary dysfunction. The authors mention that 229 postmenopausal women who did not have any obstructive coronary artery disease were measured for serum uric acid, C-reactive protein, and neutrophil count. The average age was 58 years. About 48% of women had hypertension, 5.6% had type 2 diabetes mellitus, and 61.8% had hyperlipidemia. About 59% of postmenopausal women were diagnosed with coronary endothelial dysfunction (CED). The findings of this study were as follows.

Women after menopause with CED had higher serum uric acid as compared to women after menopause without CED. Also, C-reactive protein and neutrophil count were higher in postmenopausal women with CED and it was in correlation with the high uric acid levels in these women as opposed to postmenopausal women without CED. Serum uric acid levels are linked to postmenopausal women with coronary dysfunction and this may be associated with inflammation. The study suggests a link between serum uric acid and coronary dysfunction in women with menopause.

CONCLUSION

Menopause can significantly increase the risk of gout in women due to hormonal changes and associated factors. However, with proper lifestyle adjustments, dietary changes, and medical management, the risk and impact of gout can be effectively minimized. It is essential for postmenopausal women to work closely with their healthcare providers to monitor and manage their risk factors for gout.

SUGGESTED READINGS

1. Cho SK, Winkler CA, Lee SJ, Chang Y, Ryu S. The prevalence of hyperuricemia sharply increases from the late menopausal transition stage in middle-aged women. J Clin Med. 2019;8(3):296.
2. Hak AE, Choi HK. Menopause, postmenopausal hormone use and serum uric acid levels in US women–the Third National Health and Nutrition Examination Survey. Arthritis Res Ther. 2008;10:1-7.
3. Alkadhim HK, Mehsen JT, Hasan MA. Prevalence of joint diseases in postmenopausal women. Indian J Foren Med Toxicol. 2019;13(4):636.
4. Wingrove CS, Walton C, Stevenson JC. The effect of menopause on serum uric acid levels in non-obese healthy women. Metabolism. 1998;47(4):435-8.
5. Kang S, Kwon D, Lee J, Chung YJ, Kim MR, Namkung J, et al. Association between serum uric acid levels and bone mineral density in postmenopausal women: A cross-sectional and longitudinal study. Healthcare (Basel). 20219(12):1681.
6. Hak AE, Curhan GC, Grodstein F, Choi HK. Menopause, postmenopausal hormone use and risk of incident gout. Ann Rheum Dis. 2010;69(7):1305-9.
7. Prasad M, Matteson EL, Herrmann J, Gulati R, Rihal CS, Lerman LO, et al. Uric acid is associated with inflammation, coronary microvascular dysfunction, and adverse outcomes in postmenopausal women. Hypertension. 2017;69(2):236-42.

CHAPTER 5

Application of Local Heat and Massage in Gout-affected Joints

Shivam Mehra, Kamal Mehra, Prakash Samant, Sachin Yaswant Kale, Pramod Bhor

INTRODUCTION

Gout is a form of inflammatory arthritis that results in joint pain and swelling, typically in the form of flares lasting 1–2 weeks. It occurs when the body's urate levels become elevated over an extended period, leading to the formation of needle-shaped crystals in and around the affected joint. This process triggers inflammation and arthritis in the joint. Elevated urate levels in the body can occur when the body produces an excess of urate or removes too little of it.

WHY IS HEAT THERAPY NOT RECOMMENDED?

Using hot fermentation (heat therapy) on gout-affected joints is generally not recommended, especially during an acute gout flare-up, for several reasons:
- *Increased inflammation*:
  - *Heat can exacerbate inflammation*: Applying heat to an already inflamed joint can increase blood flow to the area, potentially making inflammation and swelling worse. Gout attacks involve intense inflammation due to the deposition of uric acid crystals in the joint, and adding heat can intensify this inflammatory reaction.

- *Increased pain*:
  - *Potential for increased pain*: The additional inflammation caused by heat can lead to more severe pain. Gout pain is often described as excruciating, and any factor that intensifies inflammation can make the pain more unbearable.
- *Swelling and fluid accumulation*:
  - *Heat can lead to fluid accumulation*: Increased blood flow to the area can cause more fluid to accumulate in the joint, leading to increased swelling. This can limit joint mobility and further aggravate the discomfort associated with gout.
- *Potential for joint damage*:
  - *Risk of further damage*: Prolonged inflammation can damage the joint and surrounding tissues. Using heat may prolong the inflammatory process, potentially leading to more damage over time.
- *Masking symptoms*:
  - *Temporary relief but long-term harm*: While heat might provide temporary relief by relaxing muscles and improving circulation, it can mask the symptoms and underlying issues, leading to delayed appropriate treatment and possible worsening of the condition.

MECHANISMS BY WHICH HEAT CAN INCREASE GOUT PAIN

- *Increased inflammation*: Gout is an inflammatory condition characterized by the deposition of uric acid crystals in joints, leading to intense inflammation. Heat can exacerbate this inflammation by dilating blood vessels and increasing blood flow to the area, which can worsen swelling and pain.
- *Enhanced sensitivity*: Heat can increase the sensitivity of nerve endings in the affected area. This heightened sensitivity can amplify the perception of pain.

- *Crystal solubility and activity*: Heat can affect the solubility and activity of uric acid crystals, potentially making them more reactive and irritating to joint tissues. This can lead to increased pain and discomfort.

While heat might seem like a comforting option for pain relief, it can actually increase gout pain by exacerbating inflammation and sensitivity in the affected area. Cold therapy is generally the preferred method for managing acute gout pain and inflammation.

RECOMMENDED ALTERNATIVES

For managing gout pain and inflammation, consider these alternatives instead of heat therapy:

- *Cold therapy*:
  - *Use cold packs*: Applying ice packs to the affected joint can help reduce inflammation, swelling, and pain. Use for 15–20 minutes several times a day, ensuring to protect the skin with a cloth or towel.
- *Rest*:
  - *Rest the affected joint*: Avoid putting stress on the inflamed joint. Resting helps to reduce irritation and allows the inflammation to subside.
- *Medications*:
  - *Anti-inflammatory drugs*: Nonsteroidal anti-inflammatory drugs (NSAIDs) like ibuprofen or prescription medications specifically for gout (e.g., colchicine or corticosteroids) can help manage pain and inflammation.
  - *Uric acid-lowering medications*: Long-term medications such as allopurinol or febuxostat may be prescribed to reduce uric acid levels and prevent future attacks.
- *Hydration*:
  - *Stay hydrated*: Drinking plenty of water helps to dilute uric acid in the blood and promote its excretion through urine.

- *Lifestyle and dietary changes*:
  - *Low-purine diet*: Avoid foods high in purines, such as red meat, organ meats, and certain seafood, which can increase uric acid levels.
  - *Weight management*: Maintain a healthy weight to reduce the strain on your joints and lower the risk of gout attacks.

MECHANISMS OF COLD THERAPY IN GOUT RELIEF

Cold therapy, also known as cryotherapy, is a common and effective method for relieving pain and inflammation associated with gout. Here is how cold therapy helps:

- *Vasoconstriction*: Cold therapy causes blood vessels to constrict (vasoconstriction), which reduces blood flow to the affected area. This helps decrease swelling and inflammation by limiting the accumulation of fluids and inflammatory cells in the joint.
- *Numbing effect*: The cold numbs the nerve endings in the affected area, reducing the sensation of pain. This analgesic effect can provide significant relief from the intense pain of a gout attack.
- *Reduced metabolic rate*: Cold temperatures slow down the metabolic rate of cells, which can reduce the production of inflammatory mediators. This can help in controlling the inflammatory response in the affected joint.
- *Decreased muscle spasms*: Cold therapy can help relax muscles around the affected joint, reducing muscle spasms and associated pain.
- *Slows down uric acid crystal activity*: Cold can help to stabilize uric acid crystals, making them less reactive and reducing their ability to irritate the joint tissues.

HOW TO APPLY COLD THERAPY FOR GOUT?

Cold packs: Use a cold pack or ice pack wrapped in a towel. Apply it to the affected joint for 15–20 minutes at a time. Do not apply ice directly to the skin to avoid frostbite.

- *Frozen vegetables*: A bag of frozen peas or corn can be used as a makeshift ice pack. Again, wrap it in a towel before applying it to the skin.
- *Ice bath*: For affected feet or hands, an ice bath can be effective. Fill a basin with cold water and ice, and immerse the affected area for short periods (10–15 minutes).
- *Frequency*: Apply cold therapy several times a day, particularly during the first 48 hours of a gout attack when inflammation and pain are at their peak.

PRECAUTIONS

- *Avoid direct skin contact*: Always use a barrier, like a towel, between the ice pack and your skin to prevent frostbite.
- *Limit application time*: Do not apply cold therapy for > 20 minutes at a time to avoid skin and tissue damage.
- *Monitor skin condition*: Check the skin regularly for any signs of ice burn or excessive redness. If any adverse effects are noticed, stop the cold therapy immediately.

CONCLUSION

Cold therapy is an effective method for managing the pain and inflammation associated with gout. By reducing blood flow, numbing the area, decreasing the metabolic rate, and stabilizing uric acid crystals, cold therapy provides significant relief during acute gout attacks. Always follow proper application techniques and precautions to ensure safe and effective treatment. Always consult with a healthcare provider for personalized advice and treatment options tailored to your specific condition and health status.

SUGGESTED READINGS

1. Schnitker MA. A History of the Treatment of Gout. Bull Hist Med. 1936;4:89.
2. Schlesinger N, Detry MA, Holland BK, Baker DG, Beutler AM, Rull M, et al. Local ice therapy during bouts of acute gouty arthritis. J Rheumatol. 2002;29(2):331-4.
3. Kurniasari MD, Monsen KA, Weng SF, Yang CY, Tsai HT. Cold water immersion directly and mediated by alleviated pain to promote quality of life in Indonesian with gout arthritis: A community-based randomized controlled trial. Biol Res Nurs. 2022;24(2):245-58.
4. Li HD, Wei X. Non-drug therapies for the treatment of acute gouty arthritis. TMR Non-Drug Therapy. 2019;2(4):136-41.

CHAPTER **6**

Who is the Biggest Culprit for Gout: Alcohol or Protein-rich Foods or Both?

Aditya Gupta, Vishal Kumar

INTRODUCTION

Gouty arthritis is characterized by rapid, sudden attacks of pain, redness, and tenderness in joints. It occurs due to the deposition of uric acid crystals in the joints. Uric acid crystals are precipitated by hyperuricemia. Uric acid is a metabolic byproduct of purine metabolism and its crystallization in joints leads to the clinical manifestations of gout triggering intense inflammation and pain. Diet plays an important role in manifestation of gout, with certain dietary components like alcohols and proteins exacerbating the condition. Studies have provided substantial evidence supporting the association between alcohol, proteins, and gout risk. A study published in the American Journal of Clinical Nutrition found that purine-rich foods, especially meats and seafood, increased the risk of gout in men. Another study highlighted the significant impact of alcohol consumption on gout risk, emphasizing the need for dietary interventions to manage hyperuricemia. This article aims to explore and compare the roles of alcohol and proteins in gout, examining their biochemical mechanisms, epidemiological evidence, and clinical implications. Furthermore, it will discuss dietary strategies and recommendations for individuals with gout to effectively manage their condition.

Biochemical Basis of Gout

Both alcohol and high-purine protein ingestion leads to increased uric acid levels through different mechanisms. Alcohol increases uric acid production and decreases its excretion. Proteins rich in purines directly elevate uric acid levels through increased intake. Alcohol produces immediate and pronounced effects to its ingestion compared to protein intake which causes hyperuricemia over time only with regular consumption. To understand why alcohol and proteins are avoided in gout, it is essential to grasp the underlying biochemical mechanisms:

- *Uric acid production and excretion*: Uric acid is a waste product formed from the breakdown of purines. Uric acid is excreted through the kidneys and hence, renal failure can also cause hyperuricemia. Hyperuricemia can be caused by increased uric acid production or decreased excretion.
- *Crystallization*: Uric acid when present in increased amounts crystallizes to form sharp, needle-like crystals in the joints and surrounding tissues leading to intense pain and inflammation which are characteristic of gout.

WHY ALCOHOL IS AVOIDED IN GOUT?

Epidemiological studies have consistently demonstrated a positive association between alcohol consumption and the risk of gout. A meta-analysis published in the Clinical Rheumatology found that higher alcohol intake, particularly beer and spirits, was significantly associated with an increased risk of gout. The study noted a dose–response relationship, where higher quantities of alcohol consumed were linked to a greater risk of developing gout.

It has been shown by a study published in The Lancet that beer and spirits significantly increased the risk of gout compared to wine. They also noted that the risk was directly proportional to the quantity of alcohol consumed.

It has been evident through studies in literature that beer has the strongest association with gout, followed by spirits, while moderate wine consumption did not show a significant increase in risk.

- *Increased uric acid production*: Alcohol has high levels of purines. Beer is rich in guanosine—a type of purine that significantly increases uric acid production when metabolized. Purines are present in varying amounts in alcoholic beverages and are metabolized into uric acid. Regular consumption of beer and spirits has been shown to elevate uric acid levels more than other types of alcohol, such as wine.
- *Decreased uric acid excretion*: Alcohol can impair the kidneys' ability to excrete uric acid effectively. Ethanol is metabolized to acetaldehyde and acetate. Acetate leads to increased competition with uric acid for excretion by the kidneys, leading to reduced excretion of uric acid.
- *Dehydration*: Alcohol has diuretic properties and can lead to dehydration. Dehydration causes impaired excretion of uric acid as the kidneys prioritize water reabsorption over the excretion of waste products by reducing renal blood flow and glomerular filtration rate. This results in higher blood concentrations of uric acid, increasing the risk of crystal formation in the joints. Alcohol inhibits the release of antidiuretic hormone (ADH), contributing to diuresis and dehydration.
- *Inflammatory response*: Alcohol consumption can trigger an inflammatory response in the body leading to exacerbation of gout, leading to more frequent and severe attacks. Chronic alcoholism is associated with metabolic syndrome, which includes conditions such as obesity, hypertension, and insulin.

WHY CERTAIN PROTEINS ARE AVOIDED IN GOUT?

Not all but some proteins lead to gout. Research on the impact of protein-rich foods on gout has produced varied results. A study in the New England Journal of Medicine found that increased consumption of red meat and seafood increased the risk of gout, while dairy products reduced the risk. The study emphasized the importance of dietary composition and the type of protein consumed.

Studies have proved that high-purine foods contribute to gout but their impact is *less significant* than that of alcohol. It is recommended to have a balanced diet with moderate purine intake with emphasis on low-purine protein sources.

- *Purine content*: Protein-rich foods, especially of animal origin, contain varying levels of purines. Red meats, organ meats (such as liver and kidneys), and certain seafood (like sardines, anchovies, shellfish, and mussels) are high in purine. These foods can lead to increased production of uric acid. Purines are nitrogenous compounds found in various foods and their metabolism results in the production of uric acid.
- *Animal versus plant proteins*: Not all protein-rich foods have the same impact on uric acid levels. Animal proteins have high purine levels compared to plant proteins. However, dairy products, despite being animal-based, are low in purines and have been shown to have a protective effect against gout. Low-fat dairy products can help lower uric acid levels and reduce the risk of gout attacks. Plant-based proteins, such as legumes (e.g., beans and lentils), nuts, and tofu, are generally lower in purines and are considered safer choices for individuals with gout.
- *Moderation and variety*: Increased consumption of food rich in purines can cause gout. However, limited consumption and a balanced diet can mitigate their impact.

Including a variety of protein sources, such as lean meats, poultry, fish, and plant-based proteins (like beans, lentils, and tofu), in diet can help maintain a healthy diet without significantly increasing the risk of gout. The impact is influenced by overall dietary patterns and individual factors such as genetics, metabolism, and comorbidities.

COMPARING ALCOHOL AND PROTEIN-RICH FOODS

Mechanisms of Impact

Alcohol affects uric acid levels through multiple mechanisms, including increased production, impaired excretion, and dehydration. Its impact is immediate and direct, often leading to rapid spikes in uric acid levels and triggering acute gout attacks.

In contrast, the impact of protein-rich foods on uric acid levels depends on their purine content and the overall dietary pattern. While high-purine foods can increase uric acid production, their effect is more gradual and can be managed through moderation and a balanced diet.

Risk Factors and Frequency

Alcohol consumption, particularly in large quantities, is a significant risk factor for gout. Studies have shown that individuals who consume beer or spirits regularly have a higher risk of developing gout compared to those who consume wine or abstain from alcohol. The frequency and quantity of alcohol consumption play a crucial role in this increased risk.

Protein-rich foods, when consumed in moderation, do not pose the same level of risk as alcohol. The frequency and quantity of high-purine food intake can be controlled more easily, and incorporating low-purine protein sources can further reduce the risk of gout.

Long-term Health Implications

Chronic alcohol consumption has broader health implications beyond gout, including liver disease, cardiovascular problems, and an increased risk of certain cancers. The long-term health effects of excessive alcohol consumption make it a more concerning factor for overall health.

While a diet high in purines can contribute to gout, it can be managed through dietary adjustments. A balanced diet that includes a variety of protein sources, along with other healthy foods can support overall health without significantly increasing the risk of gout.

DIETARY STRATEGIES FOR MANAGING GOUT

Limiting Alcohol Consumption

For individuals with gout, it is crucial to limit alcohol consumption. This involves reducing or avoiding beer and spirits, which have the highest impact on uric acid levels. Moderate wine consumption may be permissible but should still be approached with caution. Complete abstinence from alcohol may be necessary for those who experience frequent gout attacks.

Moderating Purine Intake

Managing gout through diet involves moderating the intake of high-purine foods. This means limiting the consumption of red meats, organ meats, and certain seafood. Instead, individuals should focus on low-purine protein sources such as:

- *Dairy products*: Low-fat dairy products can help lower uric acid levels.
- *Plant-based proteins*: Beans, lentils, and tofu are excellent sources of protein with lower purine content.
- *Lean meats and poultry*: Consuming these in moderation can provide necessary protein without significantly increasing purine intake.

Hydration and Healthy Lifestyle

Adequate hydration is vital for managing gout. Drinking plenty of water helps the kidneys excrete uric acid more effectively, reducing the risk of crystal formation. A healthy lifestyle, including regular exercise, maintaining a healthy weight, and managing other health conditions (such as hypertension and diabetes), can further support gout management.

CONCLUSION

In the debate over whether alcohol or protein-rich foods are the bigger culprits for gout, alcohol emerges as the more immediate and significant risk factor. Its impact on uric acid levels is multifaceted and often more pronounced, making it a primary concern for individuals with gout. Protein-rich foods, while also contributing to gout, can be managed more effectively through dietary choices and moderation.

For those at risk of gout or seeking to manage the condition, it is essential to limit alcohol consumption, especially beer and spirits, and adopt a balanced diet that includes low-purine protein sources. By making informed dietary choices and maintaining a healthy lifestyle, individuals can reduce their risk of gout attacks and improve their overall well-being.

SUGGESTED READINGS

1. Jin M, Yang F, Yang I, Yin Y, Luo JJ, Wang H, et al. Uric acid, hyperuricemia and vascular diseases. Front Biosci (Landmark Ed). 2012;17(2):656-69.
2. Belanger MJ, Wee CC, Mukamal KJ, Miller ER, Sacks FM, Appel LJ, et al. Effects of dietary macronutrients on serum urate: results from the OmniHeart trial. Am J Clin Nutr. 2021;113(6):1593-9.
3. Vedder D, Walrabenstein W, Heslinga M, de Vries R, Nurmohamed M, van Schaardenburg D, et al. Dietary interventions for gout and effect on cardiovascular risk factors: A systematic review. Nutrients. 2019;11(12):2955.

4. Syed AAS, Fahira A, Yang Q, Chen J, Li Z, Chen H, et al. The relationship between alcohol consumption and gout: A Mendelian randomization study. Genes (Basel). 2022;13(4):557.
5. Wang M, Jiang X, Wu W, Zhang D. A meta-analysis of alcohol consumption and the risk of gout. Clin Rheumatol. 2013;32(11):1641-8.
6. Choi HK, Atkinson K, Karlson EW, Willett W, Curhan G. Alcohol intake and risk of incident gout in men: a prospective study. Lancet. 2004;363(9417):1277-81.
7. Rho YH, Zhu Y, Choi HK. The epidemiology of uric acid and fructose. Semin Nephrol. 2011;31(5):410-9.
8. Zhang Y, Chen S, Yuan M, Xu Y, Xu H. Gout and Diet: A Comprehensive Review of Mechanisms and Management. Nutrients. 2022;14(17):3525.
9. Kushiyama A, Nakatsu Y, Matsunaga Y, Yamamotoya T, Mori K, Ueda K, et al. Role of uric acid metabolism-related inflammation in the pathogenesis of metabolic syndrome components such as atherosclerosis and nonalcoholic steatohepatitis. Mediators Inflamm. 2016;2016:8603164.
10. Jakše B, Jakše B, Pajek M, Pajek J. Uric acid and plant-based nutrition. Nutrients. 2019;11(8):1736.
11. Yokose C, McCormick N, Choi HK. The role of diet in hyperuricemia and gout. Curr Opin Rheumatol. 2021;33(2):135-44.

CHAPTER 7

Idiopathic Retrocalcaneal Pain and Heel Pain: Is it Gout?

Prakash Samant, Arvind J Vatkar, Sachin Yaswant Kale, Shivam Mehra, Sunil Shetty, Pramod Bhor

INTRODUCTION

Idiopathic retrocalcaneal pain and heel pain are common complaints that can significantly affect mobility and quality of life (**Fig. 1**). These conditions can arise from various causes, including gout. This chapter explores the relationship between idiopathic retrocalcaneal pain, heel pain, and gout, providing practical diagnostic and management strategies.

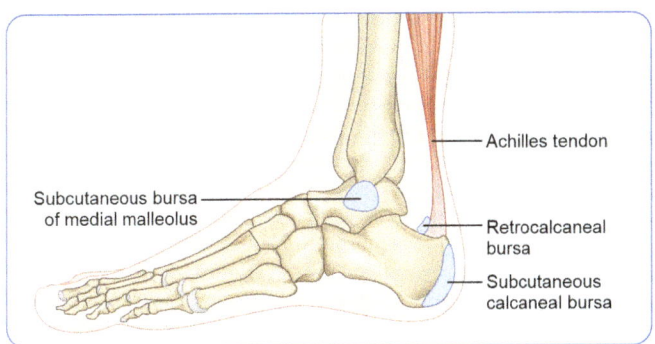

Fig. 1: Anatomy of the heel and retrocalcaneal area.

UNDERSTANDING HEEL PAIN AND RETROCALCANEAL PAIN

- *Heel pain*: General pain located around the heel.
- *Retrocalcaneal pain*: Pain specifically behind the heel, near the Achilles tendon.

There could be multiple causes of heel and retrocalcaneal pain **(Table 1)**.

GOUT AND ITS MANIFESTATIONS

Gout is a type of inflammatory arthritis caused by the deposition of uric acid crystals in joints and surrounding tissues. While it commonly affects the big toe, it can also impact other joints, including the heel. Following are the symptoms of heel and retrocalcaneal pain **(Table 2)**.

DIAGNOSTIC FLOWCHART: DETERMINING THE CAUSE OF HEEL AND RETROCALCANEAL PAIN (FLOWCHART 1 AND BOX 1)

Flowchart 2 helps in systematically determining whether heel or retrocalcaneal pain is due to gout or another condition.

MANAGEMENT OF GOUT-RELATED HEEL PAIN

There are various ways of management of gout as described in **(Table 3)**.

Table 1: Common causes of heel pain and retrocalcaneal pain.

Condition	Description	Symptoms	Diagnosis	Treatment
Plantar fasciitis	Inflammation of the plantar fascia, a thick band of tissue that runs across the bottom of the foot	Heel pain, especially in the morning or after rest	Clinical examination, ultrasound, and MRI	Rest, ice, stretching exercises, orthotics, and NSAIDs
Achilles tendinitis	Inflammation of the Achilles tendon, usually due to overuse	Pain and stiffness along the Achilles tendon, swelling	Physical examination, ultrasound, and MRI	Rest, ice, compression, elevation, and physical therapy
Heel spurs	Bony growths on the underside of the heel bone, often associated with plantar fasciitis	Chronic heel pain, especially while walking or standing	X-rays, physical examination	Rest, ice, orthotics, physical therapy, surgery (rare)
Bursitis	Inflammation of the bursa (a small sac of fluid) at the back of the heel (retrocalcaneal bursitis)	Swelling, warmth, pain at the back of the heel	Physical examination, MRI, and ultrasound	Rest, ice, NSAIDs, corticosteroid injections, and footwear changes
Sever's disease	Inflammation of the growth plate in the heel, common in growing children and adolescents	Heel pain in children, especially during physical activity	Physical examination, X-rays	Rest, ice, NSAIDs, heel pads, and stretching exercises

Continued

Continued

Condition	Description	Symptoms	Diagnosis	Treatment
Tarsal tunnel syndrome	Compression of the tibial nerve as it travels through the tarsal tunnel near the ankle	Burning, tingling, and pain in the heel and arch	Nerve conduction studies, MRI, physical examination	Rest, ice, NSAIDs, orthotics, and surgery (if severe)
Stress fractures	Small cracks in the heel bone due to repetitive stress or overuse	Deep pain in the heel, worsening with activity	X-rays, MRI, and bone scan	Rest, immobilization, gradual return to activity
Rheumatoid arthritis	Autoimmune condition causing inflammation of the joints, including those in the feet and heels	Chronic pain, swelling, stiffness in the heel and joints	Blood tests, X-rays, and physical examination	Medications (DMARDs and NSAIDs), physical therapy
Gout	A type of arthritis caused by the accumulation of uric acid crystals in the joints, including the heel	Sudden, severe pain, redness, and swelling in the heel	Blood tests (uric acid levels), joint fluid analysis	NSAIDs, corticosteroids, and uric acid-lowering medications
Heel pad syndrome	Degeneration or thinning of the fat pad that cushions the heel	Deep, bruise-like pain in the center of the heel	Physical examination, imaging tests (rarely needed)	Cushioned footwear, heel cups, rest, and ice

(DMARD: disease-modifying antirheumatic drug; MRI: magnetic resonance imaging; NSAID: nonsteroidal anti-inflammatory drug)

Table 2: Symptoms of gout in heel and retrocalcaneal region.

Symptom	Description
Sudden onset of severe pain	Intense, sharp pain that often starts suddenly, typically during the night or early morning
Swelling	Noticeable swelling in the heel or around the Achilles tendon area
Redness and warmth	The affected area may appear red and feel warm to the touch due to inflammation
Tenderness	Extreme tenderness in the heel, making it difficult to touch or bear weight on the affected foot
Limited range of motion	Difficulty moving the ankle or foot due to pain and swelling
Pain aggravated by movement	Pain may worsen with movement or pressure, such as walking or standing
	In chronic cases, deposits of uric acid crystals (tophi) may form lumps under the skin near the heel
Recurring attacks	Repeated episodes of similar symptoms in the same or other joints, indicative of chronic gout
Nighttime attacks	Symptoms often begin or worsen at night, disrupting sleep
Fever and malaise	In severe cases, systemic symptoms like low-grade fever and general discomfort may occur

CHAPTER 7: Idiopathic Retrocalcaneal Pain and Heel Pain: Is it Gout?

```
┌─────────────────────────────────────────────────────────┐
│  Patient presents with heel and/or retrocalcaneal pain  │
└─────────────────────────────────────────────────────────┘
                            ↓
┌─────────────────────────────────────────────────────────┐
│                   Initial assessment                    │
│  • Duration of pain                                     │
│  • Onset (sudden or gradual)                            │
│  • Activity level and changes                           │
│  • Recent injuries                                      │
│  • Medical history (gout, diabetes, arthritis)          │
│  • Location and nature of pain (sharp, dull, burning)   │
└─────────────────────────────────────────────────────────┘
                            ↓
┌─────────────────────────────────────────────────────────┐
│                  Physical examination                   │
│  • Inspect for swelling, redness, deformity             │
│  • Palpate heel, Achilles tendon, surrounding areas     │
│  • Assess range of motion and gait                      │
└─────────────────────────────────────────────────────────┘
                            ↓
┌─────────────────────────────────────────────────────────┐
│                  Symptom characteristics                │
│  • Start with symptoms                                  │
└─────────────────────────────────────────────────────────┘
```

- Ask if there's sudden, severe pain, redness, and swelling
- **Yes:** Consider **Possible Gout**
  – Perform blood tests for uric acid levels
  – Conduct joint fluid analysis
  – Manage with NSAIDs, corticosteroids, and uric acid-lowering medications
  – **No:** Proceed to the next evaluation

Morning pain or after rest:
- Does pain worsen with the first steps in the morning or after rest?
- **Yes:** Consider **Possible Plantar Fasciitis**
  – Perform a clinical exam and ultrasound for diagnosis
  – Manage with rest, ice, stretching, orthotics, and NSAIDs
  – **No:** Proceed to the next evaluation

Pain and stiffness along Achilles tendon:
- Is there pain and stiffness along the Achilles tendon?
- **Yes:** Consider **Possible Achilles Tendinitis**
  – Perform a physical exam, ultrasound, and possibly an MRI for diagnosis
  – Manage with rest, ice, compression, elevation, and physical therapy
  – **No:** Proceed to the next evaluation

Swelling and warmth at the back of the heel:
- Is there pain with swelling and warmth at the back of the heel?
- **Yes:** Consider **Possible Bursitis (Retrocalcaneal Bursitis)**
  – Perform a physical exam, MRI, and ultrasound for diagnosis
  – Manage with rest, ice, NSAIDs, corticosteroid injections, and footwear changes
  – **No:** Proceed to the next evaluation

Flowchart 1: The cause of heel and retrocalcaneal pain.

(MRI: magnetic resonance imaging; NSAID: nonsteroidal anti-inflammatory drug)

BOX 1: Differential diagnosis.

Heel pain in a growing child, especially during physical activity:
- Does the child experience heel pain, especially dining physical activity?
- Yes: Consider possible Sever's disease.
  - Conduct a clinical exam and X-rays for diagnosis
  - Manage with rest, ice, NSAIDs, heel pads, and stretching exercises
  - No: Proceed to the next evaluation

Burning, tingling pain in heel and arch:
- Is there a burning, tingling pain in the heel and arch?
- Yes: Consider possible tarsal tunnel syndrome
  - Perform nerve conduction studies and possibly an MRI for diagnosis
  - Manage with rest, ice, NSAIDs, orthotics, and surgery if severe
  - No: Proceed to the next evaluation

Deep pain in heel, worsening with activity:
- Does the pain feel deep in the heel and worsen with activity?
- Yes: Consider possible stress fracture
  - Perform X-rays, MRI, and possibly a bone scan for diagnosis
  - Manage with rest, immobilization, and a gradual return to activity
  - No: Proceed to the next evaluation

Chronic pain, swelling, stiffness in heel and other joints:
- Is there chronic pain, swelling, and stiffness in the heel and other joints?
- Yes: Consider possible rheumatoid arthritis
  - Conduct blood tests, X-rays, and a clinical examination for diagnosis
  - Manage with medications like DMARDs and NSAIDs, along with physical therapy
  - No: Proceed to the next evaluation

Deep, bruise-like pain in the center of the heel:
- Is there a deep, bruise-like pain in the center of the heel?
- Yes: Consider possible heel pad syndrome
  - Perform a clinical exam and imaging if needed for diagnosis
  - Manage with cushioned footwear, heel cups, rest, and ice
  - No: End of evaluation process

Patient history and physical examination
- Assess pain characteristics, duration, and onset
- Check for signs of inflammation (redness, warmth, swelling)

Initial laboratory tests
- Blood tests for uric acid levels
- Complete blood count (CBC) to rule out infection

Imaging studies
- X-ray to check for bone abnormalities
- Ultrasound or MRI if soft tissue involvement is suspected

Joint fluid analysis
- Aspiration of joint fluid to check for uric acid crystals
- Helps confirm gout diagnosis

Histopathology of soft tissue

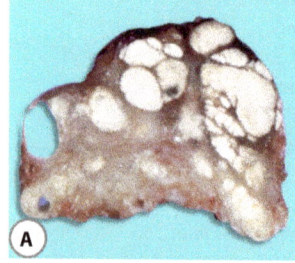 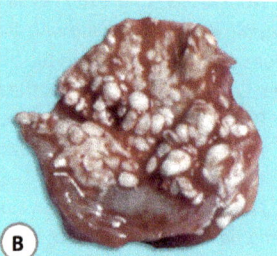

Uric acid crystal formation
Formation of MSU crystals in tophi. (A) Section through an elbow tophus showing large white MSU all-crystal-containing areas. *Image Courtesy:* F. Perez-Ruiz (B) An elbow tophus opened after surgical removal shows the corresponding white rounded nodules.
MSU: monosodium urate monohydrate
Source: Pascual E, Addadi L, Andres M, Sivera F. Mechanisms of crystal formation in gout—a structural approach. Nat Rev Rheumatol. 2015;11(12):725-30.

Differential diagnosis
- If uric acid crystals are present, diagnose as gout
- If absent, consider other causes like plantar fasciitis, Achilles tendinitis, etc.

Flowchart 2: Determining whether heel or retrocalcaneal pain is due to gout or another condition.

Table 3: Management strategies for gout in heel and retrocalcaneal region.

Management strategy	Description	Example
Medications	Pharmacological treatments to manage pain, inflammation, and uric acid levels	NSAIDs (ibuprofen and naproxen), colchicine, corticosteroids, allopurinol, and febuxostat
Rest and joint protection	Reducing stress on the affected joint to minimize pain and inflammation	Avoiding weight-bearing activities, using crutches, and wearing supportive footwear
Ice therapy	Applying cold packs to reduce inflammation and numb the area	Ice packs or cold compresses applied for 15–20 minutes several times a day
Hydration	Drinking plenty of fluids to help flush out uric acid from the body	Water, herbal teas, avoiding alcohol and sugary beverages
Dietary modifications	Changing diet to lower uric acid levels and reduce the risk of gout attacks	Low-purine diet, avoiding red meat, organ meats, certain seafood, and high-fructose foods
Weight management	Maintaining a healthy weight to reduce stress on joints and lower uric acid levels	Regular exercise, balanced diet, avoiding crash diets, and rapid weight loss
Physical therapy	Exercises to improve joint function, strength, and flexibility	Stretching, strengthening exercises, guided by a physical therapist
Topical treatments	Applying creams or gels to reduce pain and inflammation	Topical NSAIDs, capsaicin cream

Continued

Continued

Management strategy	Description	Example
Footwear adjustments	Using appropriate shoes to reduce pressure on the heel and improve comfort	Cushioned shoes, orthotic inserts, and heel pads
Monitoring and follow-up	Regular check-ups to monitor uric acid levels and adjust treatment as needed	Blood tests, follow-up appointments with a healthcare provider
Patient education	Informing patients about gout management and prevention strategies	Educational materials, support groups, counseling on lifestyle changes

CONCLUSION

Idiopathic retrocalcaneal pain and heel pain can have various causes, with gout being a significant one. Proper diagnosis involves a combination of patient history, physical examination, laboratory tests, and imaging studies. Effective management includes medication, lifestyle modifications, and regular monitoring. Understanding the potential link between these pains and gout can lead to better patient outcomes through targeted treatment strategies.

By following the diagnostic flowchart and employing appropriate management techniques, healthcare providers can effectively distinguish between gout and other causes of heel and retrocalcaneal pain, ensuring accurate diagnosis, and optimal care for patients.

SUGGESTED READINGS

1. Duran E, Bilgin E, Ertenli Aİ, Kalyoncu U. The frequency of Achilles and plantar calcaneal spurs in gout patients. Turkish Journal of Medical Sciences. 2021;51(4):1841-8.
2. Sarkar D, Hoque TM. Association of High Serum Uric Acid with Retrocalcaneal Buristis. International Journal of Medical Science and Health Research. 2019;3(3):ISSN:2581-3366.
3. Yates B. The painful foot. Merriman's Assessment of the Lower Limb. 3th. Ed. Edinburgh: Elsevier. 2009:469-98.
4. Aronow MS. Posterior heel pain (retrocalcaneal bursitis, insertional and noninsertional Achilles tendinopathy). Clinics in podiatric medicine and surgery. 2005;22(1):19-43.

CHAPTER **8**

Gout in Pregnancy

**Smruti Sachin Kale, Sumedha Shinde,
Nindiya Kapoor Mehra, Sachiti Sachin Kale**

INTRODUCTION

Hyperuricemia, a condition characterized by elevated levels of uric acid in the blood, can pose significant challenges during pregnancy. While typically associated with gout and kidney stones, hyperuricemia during pregnancy can also signal potential complications for both the mother and the developing fetus. Understanding the causes, risks, management strategies, and potential complications of hyperuricemia in pregnancy is crucial for ensuring maternal and fetal health.

UNDERSTANDING HYPERURICEMIA

Uric acid is a waste product formed from the breakdown of purines, substances found in certain foods and drinks and produced by the body. Normally, uric acid dissolves in the blood, passes through the kidneys, and is excreted in urine. Hyperuricemia occurs when there is an imbalance between uric acid production and excretion, leading to its accumulation in the blood.

SYMPTOMS OF HYPERURICEMIA

- Often asymptomatic in its early stages
- Can lead to gout, characterized by joint pain, redness, and swelling
- May cause kidney stones or renal dysfunction in severe cases

HYPERURICEMIA IN PREGNANCY: PREVALENCE AND CAUSES

Hyperuricemia is relatively uncommon in pregnant women, but certain conditions and factors can increase its occurrence:

- *Preeclampsia*: A pregnancy complication characterized by high blood pressure and signs of damage to another organ system, often the kidneys. Elevated uric acid levels are commonly associated with preeclampsia.
- *Chronic hypertension*: Preexisting high blood pressure can impair kidney function, leading to reduced uric acid excretion.
- *Obesity*: Excess body weight can increase uric acid production and decrease its excretion.
- *Renal dysfunction*: Preexisting kidney conditions or those developed during pregnancy can lead to hyperuricemia.
- *Gestational diabetes*: Insulin resistance associated with gestational diabetes can contribute to elevated uric acid levels.
- *Diet*: High intake of purine-rich foods and beverages can increase uric acid levels.

MECHANISM OF HYPERURICEMIA IN PREGNANCY

The mechanism of hyperuricemia in pregnancy is complex and involves several physiological changes and potential pathological processes. Here are the primary mechanisms:

- *Increased production of uric acid*:
  - *Increased cell turnover*: Pregnancy induces increased cell proliferation and turnover, leading to higher production of uric acid.
  - *Oxidative stress*: Elevated levels of oxidative stress during pregnancy can increase uric acid production as a byproduct of purine metabolism.
- *Decreased renal clearance*:
  - *Reduced kidney function*: Pregnancy places additional strain on the kidneys, which can reduce their ability to filter and excrete uric acid effectively.
  - *Hormonal changes*: Hormonal alterations, especially increased levels of estrogen and progesterone, can affect renal blood flow and glomerular filtration rate, leading to decreased excretion of uric acid.
- *Hemodynamic changes*:
  - *Increased blood volume*: Pregnancy results in increased blood volume and cardiac output, which can affect kidney function and uric acid clearance.
  - *Volume expansion*: As blood volume expands, the kidneys may initially excrete more uric acid. However, as the pregnancy progresses, the increased blood volume may lead to relative hypoperfusion of the kidneys, reducing uric acid clearance.
- *Placental factors*:
  - *Placental dysfunction*: Poor placental function can lead to hypoxia and oxidative stress, which can increase uric acid production.
  - *Inflammatory mediators*: Placental ischemia can stimulate the release of inflammatory mediators that may interfere with uric acid metabolism.

- *Dietary factors*:
  - *Increased intake of purine-rich foods*: Pregnant women might change their diet, and an increase in foods high in purines can elevate uric acid levels.
  - *Insulin resistance*: Pregnancy-induced insulin resistance can lead to increased levels of uric acid, as insulin normally helps in the renal excretion of uric acid.

The mechanisms of hyperuricemia in pregnancy are multifactorial, involving increased production of uric acid, decreased renal clearance, hemodynamic and hormonal changes, placental factors, and dietary influences. Understanding these mechanisms is crucial for monitoring and managing hyperuricemia to prevent complications during pregnancy.

IMPACT OF HYPERURICEMIA ON PREGNANCY

Hyperuricemia during pregnancy can have significant implications for both the mother and the fetus **(Fig. 1)**.

Pathophysiological Implications

Maternal risks:
- *Preeclampsia*: Hyperuricemia is closely linked to preeclampsia. Uric acid may contribute to endothelial dysfunction, inflammation, and oxidative stress, all of which are central features of preeclampsia.
- Potential for acute kidney injury or worsening of chronic kidney disease (CKD)
- Elevated blood pressure and cardiovascular complications

Fetal risks:
- *Fetal growth restriction (FGR)*: High uric acid levels can affect placental function, leading to reduced nutrient and oxygen delivery to the fetus, causing growth restriction, that is, intrauterine growth restriction (IUGR) due to placental insufficiency.

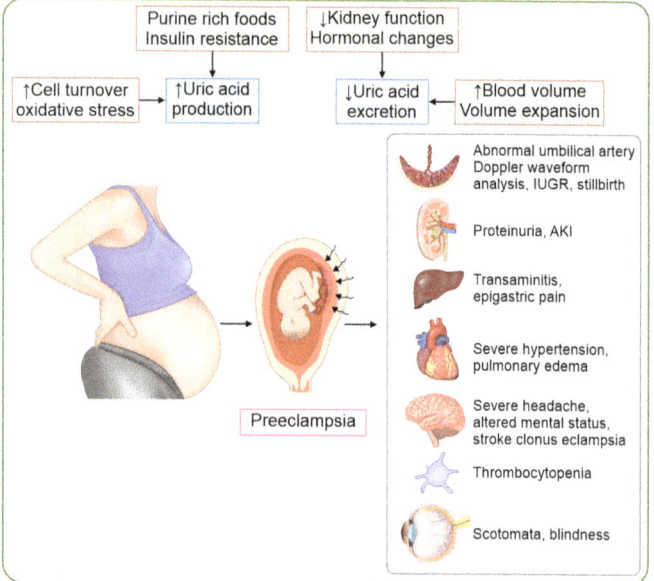

Fig. 1: Hyperuricemia in pregnancy can cause preeclampsia and intrauterine growth restriction (IUGR).
(AKI: acute kidney injury)

- Preterm birth
- Low birth weight
- Increased risk of perinatal morbidity and mortality

CLINICAL SCENARIOS OF HYPERURICEMIA IN PREGNANCY

Hyperuricemia in pregnancy can present in various clinical scenarios, often associated with specific pregnancy-related complications. Here are some examples:
- *Preeclampsia*:
  - *Case example*: A 30-year-old pregnant woman at 28 weeks of gestation presents with high blood pressure

(150/95 mm Hg) and proteinuria (2+ on a dipstick). Her serum uric acid level is found to be 7.5 mg/dL (normal range: 3.5–5.9 mg/dL for women). She is diagnosed with preeclampsia, and the elevated uric acid level is used as a marker for the severity of her condition.

- *Gestational hypertension*:
  - *Case example*: A 25-year-old woman at 32 weeks of gestation presents with new-onset hypertension (140/90 mm Hg) without proteinuria. Her serum uric acid level is elevated at 6.8 mg/dL. She is monitored closely for the potential development of preeclampsia, as hyperuricemia in gestational hypertension can indicate a higher risk of progression to preeclampsia.
- *Fetal growth restriction*:
  - *Case example*: A 29-year-old woman at 30 weeks of gestation is found to have a fetus with growth measurements below the 10th percentile for gestational age. Her serum uric acid level is 7.0 mg/dL. Elevated uric acid in the context of FGR suggests possible placental insufficiency and increased oxidative stress, prompting more frequent monitoring and potential early delivery.
- *Insulin resistance and gestational diabetes*:
  - *Case example*: A 34-year-old pregnant woman with a body mass index (BMI) of 32 presents at 28 weeks of gestation with a positive glucose tolerance test, indicating gestational diabetes. Her serum uric acid level is elevated at 6.5 mg/dL. Hyperuricemia in this context reflects the underlying insulin resistance and metabolic changes associated with gestational diabetes.
- *Chronic kidney disease exacerbated by pregnancy*:
  - *Case example*: A 35-year-old woman with a history of mild CKD becomes pregnant. At 24 weeks of gestation, her serum creatinine rises from baseline levels, and her serum uric acid level is 8.0 mg/dL. The pregnancy exacerbates her underlying kidney condition, leading to reduced clearance of uric acid and hyperuricemia.

- *Obesity-related hyperuricemia*:
  - *Case example*: A 28-year-old pregnant woman with a BMI of 35 presents at 26 weeks of gestation for a routine check-up. Her serum uric acid level is 7.2 mg/dL. She does not have hypertension or proteinuria, but her obesity contributes to elevated uric acid levels, warranting close monitoring for potential complications like gestational hypertension or preeclampsia.

These examples illustrate how hyperuricemia can manifest in different pregnancy-related conditions. Monitoring serum uric acid levels in pregnant women, especially those with risk factors, can provide valuable information for the early detection and management of potential complications.

MANAGEMENT OF HYPERURICEMIA IN PREGNANCY

Managing hyperuricemia during pregnancy involves a combination of lifestyle modifications, careful medication use, and regular monitoring to ensure the health and well-being of both mother and baby.

Lifestyle Modifications

- *Diet*:
  - Avoid purine-rich foods such as red meat, organ meats, and certain seafood.
  - Limit intake of high-fructose corn syrup and sugary beverages.
  - Emphasize a balanced diet with plenty of fruits, vegetables, whole grains, and low-fat dairy products.
- *Hydration*:
  - Ensure adequate fluid intake to help dilute uric acid and promote its excretion.
- *Weight management*:
  - Maintain a healthy weight through a balanced diet and pregnancy-safe exercise.

Medication

Medication use during pregnancy must be carefully considered due to potential risks to the developing fetus. While many medications used to manage hyperuricemia in nonpregnant individuals are contraindicated during pregnancy, some options may be used under medical supervision:

- *Corticosteroids*:
    - May be used to manage acute conditions associated with hyperuricemia, such as preeclampsia.
- *Antihypertensive medications*:
    - Used to manage blood pressure, which can be critical in cases of hyperuricemia associated with preeclampsia or chronic hypertension.

Monitoring and Medical Support

Regular monitoring by healthcare professionals is essential for pregnant women with hyperuricemia:

- *Blood tests*:
    - Regular monitoring of uric acid levels and kidney function
- *Prenatal care*:
    - Frequent prenatal visits to monitor maternal and fetal health
- *Specialist consultation*:
    - Involvement of a nephrologist or a maternal–fetal medicine specialist for comprehensive management
- *Potential complications*:
    - Hyperuricemia during pregnancy can lead to several complications if not properly managed.
- *Preeclampsia*:
    - Elevated uric acid levels are a marker for preeclampsia, which can progress to eclampsia, a life-threatening condition.
- *Kidney damage*:
    - Persistent hyperuricemia can cause or exacerbate renal dysfunction.

- *Fetal complications*: Intrauterine growth restriction, preterm birth, and low birth weight can result from placental insufficiency associated with hyperuricemia.

CONCLUSION

Hyperuricemia in pregnancy presents significant challenges that require careful management to protect both maternal and fetal health. Through lifestyle modifications, regular medical monitoring, and appropriate treatment strategies, pregnant women with hyperuricemia can minimize risks and improve outcomes. Continued research and better understanding of hyperuricemia's impact on pregnancy will further enhance care for this vulnerable population.

SUGGESTED READINGS

1. Ahmed MM, Saad NE, Abbas SM, El Azizi TM, El Sayed I. Elevated uric acid in gestational diabetes and its risk on pregnancy outcomes. SAGE Open Med. 2024;12:20503121241241934.
2. Powers RW, Bodnar LM, Ness RB, Cooper KM, Gallaher MJ, Frank MP, et al. Uric acid concentrations in early pregnancy among preeclamptic women with gestational hyperuricemia at delivery. Am J Obstet Gynecol. 2006;194(1):160.
3. Tan J, Fei H, Chen L, Zhu X. The association of hyperuricemia and maternal and fetal outcomes among pregnant women: a meta-analysis. J Matern Fetal Neonatal Med. 2023;36(1):2212830.
4. Laughon SK, Catov J, Powers RW, Roberts JM, Gandley RE. First trimester uric acid and adverse pregnancy outcomes. Am J Hypertens. 2011;24(4):489-95.
5. Lüscher BP, Schoeberlein A, Surbek DV, Baumann MU. Hyperuricemia during pregnancy leads to a preeclampsia-like phenotype in mice. Cells. 2022;11(22):3703.

CHAPTER **9**

Gout in Spine

*Arvind J Vatkar, Sachin Yashwant Kale,
Vishal Kumar, Aditya Gupta*

INTRODUCTION

Hyperuricemia, characterized by elevated levels of uric acid in the blood, is a well-recognized risk factor for gout, a form of inflammatory arthritis. However, its role extends beyond the classic presentation of gout, implicating various other musculoskeletal conditions, including those affecting the spine. This chapter explores the correlation between hyperuricemia and spinal disorders examining the underlying mechanisms, clinical manifestations, diagnostic challenges, and management strategies.

PATHOPHYSIOLOGY OF HYPERURICEMIA

Hyperuricemia can lead to the formation of monosodium urate (MSU) crystals, which are known to induce a potent inflammatory response. This inflammatory process can exacerbate preexisting spinal conditions or even contribute to the development of new spinal pathologies. Chronic inflammation is a well-established factor in spinal disorders such as disk degeneration and spinal osteoarthritis. The presence of urate crystals in spinal joints and tissues can perpetuate inflammation, thus worsening these conditions.

Uric acid is the end product of purine metabolism in humans. Hyperuricemia occurs when there is an imbalance between uric acid production and excretion. Factors contributing to this imbalance include:

- *Increased production*:
  - *Dietary factors*: Diets high in purines (e.g., red meat and seafood) significantly increase uric acid production.
  - *Increased nucleic acid turnover*: Conditions such as hematological malignancies and rapid cell turnover increase uric acid production.
- *Decreased excretion*:
  - *Renal insufficiency*: Impaired kidney function reduces the excretion of uric acid.
  - *Medications*: Diuretics and low-dose aspirin decrease uric acid excretion by the kidneys.

MECHANISMS LINKING HYPERURICEMIA TO SPINAL DISORDERS

The correlation between hyperuricemia and spinal disorders is multifaceted. Several mechanisms have been proposed to explain this relationship:

- *Crystal deposition*: MSU crystals can deposit in the spinal structures, including intervertebral disks, facet joints, and spinal ligaments, leading to local inflammation, bone erosion, and spinal cord or nerve root compression. The deposition of urate crystals in the spinal joints can mimic other spinal disorders, complicating the diagnostic process and treatment strategies. Clinical manifestations of spinal gout can range from localized pain and stiffness to severe neurological deficits, depending on the location and extent of crystal deposition.
- *Inflammatory cascade*: Hyperuricemia triggers an inflammatory response, with elevated levels of cytokines such as interleukin-1β (IL-1β) and tumor necrosis factor-alpha (TNF-α). These inflammatory mediators can contribute

to the degeneration of spinal structures and exacerbate existing spinal conditions.

- *Intervertebral disk degeneration*: Recent studies have indicated a possible link between hyperuricemia and intervertebral disk degeneration. Elevated uric acid levels can contribute to oxidative stress and inflammation within the disk tissue, accelerating the degenerative process. This degeneration often leads to chronic back pain, decreased spinal flexibility, and impaired function. Understanding this connection is crucial, as it may open new avenues for preventing or slowing down the progression of disk degeneration in hyperuricemic patients.
- *Comorbidities*: Hyperuricemia frequently coexists with other metabolic conditions such as obesity, diabetes, and hypertension, all of which are known risk factors for spinal disorders. These comorbidities can compound the adverse effects of hyperuricemia on spinal health, leading to a higher prevalence and severity of spinal problems in affected individuals. For instance, obesity increases mechanical stress on the spine, while diabetes and hypertension can contribute to vascular and neural compromise, further aggravating spinal conditions.
- *Decreased bone density*: Uric acid has a dual role in bone metabolism, with both protective antioxidant effects and detrimental pro-oxidant activities depending on its concentration. While low levels of uric acid may offer some protection against oxidative damage, high levels are associated with increased bone resorption and decreased bone density. This makes the spine more vulnerable to fractures and other structural problems, particularly in older adults or those with preexisting bone health issues.
- *Neurological manifestations*: The neurological implications of hyperuricemia extend to conditions such as spinal stenosis and other compressive neuropathies. The inflammatory response and crystal deposition in the spinal region can lead to nerve compression, resulting in

symptoms such as pain, numbness, and reduced mobility. These neurological manifestations highlight the need for clinicians to consider hyperuricemia as a potential underlying factor when diagnosing and treating spinal disorders.

CLINICAL MANIFESTATIONS

The clinical manifestations of hyperuricemia-related spinal disorders are varied and can mimic other spinal conditions. Common presentations include:
- *Acute back pain*: Sudden onset of severe back pain, potentially due to acute gouty attacks in the spine.
- *Chronic back pain*: Persistent back pain, which may be due to chronic inflammation or degenerative changes associated with hyperuricemia.
- *Neurological symptoms*: Radiculopathy, myelopathy, or cauda equina syndrome can occur if MSU crystals compress nerve roots or the spinal cord.
- *Spinal stiffness and limited mobility*: Inflammation and structural changes can lead to reduced spinal flexibility and movement.

DIAGNOSTIC CHALLENGES

Diagnosing spinal disorders related to hyperuricemia is challenging due to the nonspecific nature of symptoms and the overlap with other spinal conditions. Key diagnostic approaches include:
- *Imaging studies*:
  - *X-rays and CT scans*: May show bone erosions, tophi, or degenerative changes, but these findings are not specific to hyperuricemia.
  - *MRI*: Can detect soft tissue changes, inflammation, and tophi, especially with gadolinium enhancement.

- *Laboratory tests*:
  - *Serum uric acid levels*: Elevated uric acid levels support the diagnosis but are not definitive, as some patients with hyperuricemia-related spinal disorders may have normal uric acid levels during acute attacks.
  - *Inflammatory markers*: Elevated C-reactive protein (CRP) and erythrocyte sedimentation rate (ESR) indicate an inflammatory process but are nonspecific.
- *Definitive diagnosis*:
  - *Aspiration and analysis of synovial fluid or tophi*: Identifying MSU crystals under polarized light microscopy remains the gold standard for diagnosing gout but is often impractical for spinal involvement due to the inaccessibility of affected sites.

MANAGEMENT STRATEGIES

Management of hyperuricemia-related spinal disorders involves a combination of pharmacologic and nonpharmacologic approaches aimed at controlling hyperuricemia, reducing inflammation, and addressing spinal pathology.

- *Pharmacologic treatment*:
  - *Acute gout flares*:
    - *Nonsteroidal anti-inflammatory drugs (NSAIDs)*: First-line treatment to reduce inflammation and pain
    - *Colchicine*: Effective for acute flares, with careful dosing to avoid toxicity
    - *Corticosteroids*: Oral or intravenous, used when NSAIDs and colchicine are contraindicated or ineffective.
  - *Chronic management*:
    - *Urate-lowering therapy (ULT)*: Allopurinol or febuxostat to maintain serum uric acid levels below target thresholds, preventing crystal deposition

- **Anti-inflammatory prophylaxis**: Low-dose colchicine or NSAIDs to prevent flares during ULT initiation
- *Non-pharmacologic interventions*:
  - *Physical therapy*: Tailored exercise programs to improve mobility, strength, and function while minimizing pain
  - *Lifestyle modifications*: Dietary changes to reduce purine intake, weight management, and increased hydration to prevent hyperuricemia.
- *Surgical intervention*: Indicated in cases of severe neurological compromise or when conservative treatments fail. Surgical options may include decompression, removal of tophi, or spinal fusion, depending on the extent and location of the pathology.

CASE STUDIES AND CLINICAL OUTCOMES

Several case studies illustrate the impact of hyperuricemia on spinal disorders:
- *Case study 1*: A 60-year-old male with chronic hyperuricemia presented with lumbar radiculopathy. MRI revealed tophaceous deposits compressing the nerve roots. Management with ULT and anti-inflammatory medications resulted in significant symptom improvement.
- *Case study 2*: A 65-year-old female presented with hyperuricemia and severe cervical myelopathy. Imaging showed extensive tophi causing spinal cord compression. Surgical decompression combined with ULT led to substantial neurological recovery and pain relief.

CONCLUSION

Hyperuricemia, while primarily associated with gout, has significant implications for spinal health. The correlation between hyperuricemia and spinal disorders underscores the complex interplay between metabolic and musculoskeletal health. Recognizing this connection is vital for developing comprehensive treatment plans that address both hyperuricemia and its potential musculoskeletal complications. Elevated uric acid levels can exacerbate inflammation, contribute to disk degeneration, and increase the risk of comorbid conditions, all of which negatively impact spinal health. Its role in spinal disorders underscores the importance of recognizing and managing elevated uric acid levels to prevent and mitigate spinal complications. Through a combination of targeted pharmacologic treatments, lifestyle modifications, and when necessary, surgical interventions, effective management of hyperuricemia-related spinal disorders can be achieved, improving patient outcomes and quality of life. Ongoing research is essential to further elucidate the mechanisms and optimize therapeutic strategies for this complex and multifaceted condition.

FUTURE DIRECTIONS AND RESEARCH

Understanding the full impact of hyperuricemia on spinal health is an evolving area of research. Future studies should aim to:

- *Elucidate pathophysiological mechanisms*: Further investigate the molecular and cellular pathways linking hyperuricemia to spinal disorders.
- *Identify biomarkers*: Develop specific biomarkers to aid in the diagnosis and monitoring of hyperuricemia-related spinal conditions.
- *Optimize therapeutic strategies*: Assess the efficacy of different pharmacologic and nonpharmacologic interventions in larger, more diverse populations.
- *Explore genetic factors*: Investigate genetic predispositions that may influence the relationship between hyperuricemia and spinal disorders.

- *Longitudinal studies*: Conduct long-term studies to understand the progression and outcomes of spinal disorders in patients with hyperuricemia.

By addressing these areas, researchers and clinicians can improve the management of hyperuricemia-related spinal disorders, ultimately enhancing patient care and quality of life.

SUGGESTED READINGS

1. Dalbeth N, Merriman TR, Stamp LK. Gout. Lancet. 2016; 388(10055):2039-52.
2. Wang H, Wang J. Uric acid and inflammation in metabolic syndrome. J Inflamm Res. 2018;11:101-9.
3. Toprover M, Krasnokutsky S. Spinal gout. Rheumat Dis Clin. 2018;44(2):451-68.
4. Gerster JC, Duvoisin B. Gout and axial involvement: Clinical features and radiological signs. Rheumatology. 2001;40(2):120-4.
5. Battie MC, Videman T, Kaprio J. The twin spine study: Contributions to a changing view of disc degeneration. Spine J. 2007;7(5): 471-81.
6. Harma M. Obesity is a risk factor for low back pain and sciatica. Clin Spine Surg. 2004;17(2):107-11.
7. Veronese N, Reginster JY. Uric acid and osteoarthritis: a systematic review and meta-analysis. Eur J Int Med. 2016;34:29-36.
8. Chen LX, Schumacher HR. Gout: spine and spinal cord involvement. J Clin Rheumatol. 2008;14(3):166-8.

CHAPTER 10

Gout: The Do's and Don'ts

Vishal Kumar, Shivam Mehra, Kamal Mehra, Sunil Shetty

INTRODUCTION

Gout is a common and complex form of arthritis characterized by sudden, severe attacks of pain, swelling, redness, and tenderness in the joints. Urate crystals are formed in joints due to elevated levels of uric acid in the blood and can cause acute gout attacks. Some people manage to keep uric acid levels in control by eating less purine-rich foods like meat, seafood, as well as alcohol.

Purines break down to release uric acid. Purines are mainly endogenous, but they are also found externally in many foods that we eat. Purine-rich foods include fish, meat, seafood, etc. People who suffer from gout are advised to have a low purine-rich diet. But it is not clear exactly how effective that kind of diet is.

If people having gout adopt some healthy strategies to self-manage that include physical activity, healthy diet and healthy weight and its maintenance, they can avoid the risk of gout attacks. Managing gout effectively requires a mixture of medication, lifestyle adjustments, and dietary modifications. Following are the do's and don'ts for managing gout.

THE DO'S

Stay Hydrated

Uric acid in the blood is diluted by keeping the body hydrated. It also promotes excretion of uric acid through urine, thereby reducing the risk of crystal formation in the joints. Aim to drink at least 8–16 cups of water daily. Proper hydration also aids kidney function, which is crucial in managing uric acid levels. Additionally, staying hydrated can help prevent renal stones formation, a common complication of gout.

Follow a Low-purine Diet

Purines are metabolized to uric acid by the body. Consuming foods low in purines can help control uric acid levels. Key dietary recommendations include:
- *Fruits and vegetables*: Fruits and vegetables generally contain less purines and are rich in fiber, vitamins, and minerals. Cherries contain anthocyanins, and have been shown to have therapeutic effects in reducing uric acid levels and inflammation.
- *Whole grains*: Oatmeal, brown rice, and whole-wheat bread are low in purines and beneficial for overall health.
- *Low-fat dairy products*: These may help reduce the risk of gout attacks by lowering uric acid.

Maintain a Healthy Weight

Uric acid production is increased and its excretion is decreased in obesity. Following a healthy lifestyle through a balanced diet and regular physical activity is imperative. Gradual weight loss is recommended, as rapid weight loss can increase uric acid levels temporarily.

Take Medications as Prescribed

Adherence to prescribed medications is essential in managing gout. These medications include:

- *Urate-lowering drugs*: Medications like allopurinol and febuxostat help to reduce uric acid production.
- *Anti-inflammatory drugs*: Nonsteroidal anti-inflammatory drugs (NSAIDs), corticosteroids, and colchicine are used during acute attacks to reduce inflammation and pain.

Limit Alcohol Consumption

Alcohol increases uric acid levels and precipitates gout attacks. Beer contains high levels of purines, while spirits can interfere with uric acid metabolism. If you choose to drink, moderation is key, and wine is generally a better option than beer.

Monitor Uric Acid Levels

This can help prevent gout flare-ups and monitor the effectiveness of treatment plans. Home testing kits are available, or regular check-ups with your healthcare provider can be arranged.

Exercise Regularly

Regular physical activity helps to maintain a healthy weight and reduces stress. Low-impact exercises like walking, swimming, and cycling are particularly beneficial for people with gout as they are less likely to stress the joints. Exercise also improves overall cardiovascular health, which is important given the association between gout and cardiovascular diseases.

Consider Coffee Intake

Some studies suggest that coffee consumption may reduce the risk of developing gout. Coffee contains compounds that lower uric acid levels and have antioxidant properties. However, it is important to drink coffee in moderation and avoid adding excessive sugar or cream.

Eat More Vitamin C Rich Foods

Vitamin C has been shown to lower uric acid levels in the blood. Consider citrus fruits, strawberries, bell peppers, and broccoli into your daily diet to help manage gout.

THE DON'TS

The "don'ts" of gout management, providing evidence-based recommendations supported by scientific research and clinical guidelines.

Avoid High-purine Foods

High-purine foods should be limited or avoided to reduce uric acid levels and prevent gout attacks.

- *Red meat*: Beef, lamb, and pork are rich in purines and lead to increased chances of gout.
- *Organ meats*: Liver, kidneys, and other organ meats may increase uric acid levels significantly.
- *Seafood*: Certain types of seafood are rich in purines, including anchovies, sardines, mussels, scallops, trout, and tuna. These should be consumed sparingly or avoided to manage gout effectively.

Limit Sugary Beverages

Beverages sweetened with high-fructose corn syrup, such as sodas and some fruit drinks, lead to an increased risk of gout. Fructose can stimulate uric acid production, contributing to hyperuricemia and gout attack. It is advisable to drink water, drinks with less sugar or herbal teas to decrease the chances of gout flares.

Don't Skip Medications

Consistency in taking prescribed medications is crucial for managing gout effectively. First-line drugs include urate-lowering drugs (e.g., allopurinol and febuxostat) and anti-inflammatory drugs (e.g., NSAIDs and corticosteroids). Skipping doses or discontinuing medications without medical supervision may cause uncontrolled uric acid levels and increase incidence of gout flares.

Avoid Crash Diets

Rapid weight loss diets, also known as crash diets, can increase uric acid levels and cause sudden gout attacks. Restriction of calories during dieting can lead to disruption of the uric acid metabolism and increased formation of urate crystals in the joint. It is essential to pursue gradual and sustainable weight loss through balanced nutrition and regular physical activity to manage gout effectively.

Don't Ignore Symptoms

Prompt management of gout attacks is crucial to minimize pain and prevent joint damage. Ignoring symptoms or delaying treatment can prolong the duration and intensity of gout attacks, leading to complications such as chronic gouty arthritis and tophi formation. Early intervention with medications and lifestyle modifications can help alleviate symptoms and reduce the frequency of gout flares.

Reduce Stress

Anxiety or stress can exacerbate gout attacks and manifest symptoms in individuals with existing gout. Meditation, yoga, deep breathing exercises, and regular physical activity can decrease stress levels and improve gout symptoms. Adequate sleep and maintaining a balanced lifestyle are also essential for managing stress and minimizing the risk of gout flares.

Avoid High-dose Aspirin

High doses of aspirin can interfere with uric acid excretion potentially triggering gout flares. Alternative medications such as acetaminophen or NSAIDs are drugs of choice for pain relief.

Limit Processed Foods

High levels of salt, sugar, and unhealthy fats in processed foods can exacerbate gout symptoms. These foods may also contribute to weight gain and metabolic disturbances, further increasing the risk of gout attacks. Consuming whole, unprocessed foods such as vegetables, fruits, lean proteins, and whole grains can improve gout management and overall health.

Be Cautious with Supplements

While some dietary supplements may offer health benefits, others can potentially worsen gout symptoms or interact with medications. For example, niacin (vitamin B3) supplements can increase uric acid levels in some individuals. It is essential to consume only good-quality supplements.

Avoid Shellfish and Certain Fish

Shellfish and certain types of fish are high in purines and should be limited or avoided in a gout-friendly diet. Examples include shrimp, lobster, and sardines. Instead, choose lower-purine seafood options such as salmon, trout, and catfish to decrease the risk of gout flares.

DIET AND GOUT

An important factor in managing gout is adopting a healthy diet. Foods that are rich in purines as already mentioned like meats, seafood, certain beverages, legumes, etc., if avoided can prevent gout.

- *Role of purines in gout*: It is estimated that 70% of uric acid in the body is produced endogenously. This implies that even though a person avoids foods that are rich in purines, they can reduce the levels of uric acid in the blood by only 30%. Also, the absorption of purines from different foods is different which means that avoiding all purine-rich foods will also hamper a person's intake of a balanced diet. Further, there is not much data on the effectiveness of low purine diets **(Fig. 1)**.

  Recently, experts have started suggesting to reduce weight and maintain a healthy diet to keep gout at bay. Generally, a healthy diet focuses on the incorporation of plant-based foods, such as whole grains, vegetables, legumes, and fruits. The DASH diet (Dietary Approaches to Stop Hypertension) suggested in a study conducted in 2021 emphasizes on the fact that a plant-based protein diet reduces uric acid levels compared to a similar low-carbohydrate or low-fat diet.
  - Some foods like low-fat dairy products may even be beneficial for lowering uric acid as shown in multiple studies. Calcium-containing foods might also reduce gout attacks.
  - Certain studies also point out to the role of vitamin C in lowering uric acid levels. Consuming foods rich in vitamin C like strawberries and peppers might help prevent pain in gout.
  - Foods to include in diet when having gout:
    - Plenty of water
    - Fruits and vegetables
    - Whole grains
    - Nonmeat proteins such as low-fat dairy products, beans, and lentils
    - Lean meats and poultry

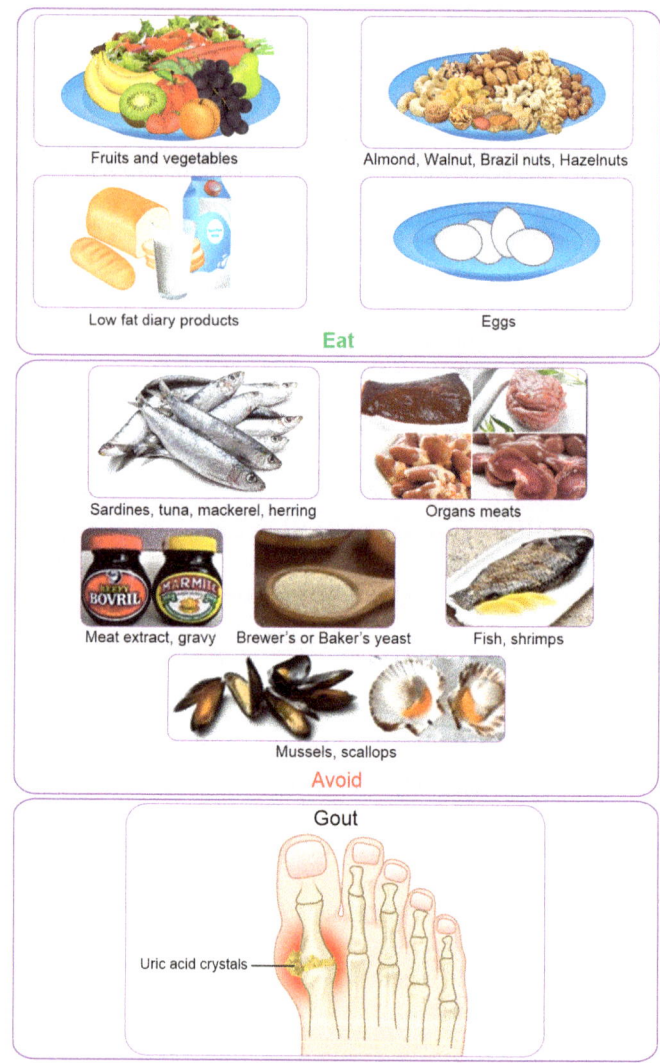

Fig. 1: Foods to eat and avoid with gout.

- Citrus fruits or foods rich in vitamin C
- Cherries or cherry juice
- *Foods to avoid with gout*:
  - Alcohol and certain foods can raise the risk of gout and trigger gout attacks.
- *Limit*:
  - Purine-rich meats (beef, lamb, and pork)
  - Purine-rich seafood (sardines and shellfish)
  - Naturally sweet fruit juices
  - Sugar and food and drinks sweetened with sugar
- *Avoid*:
  - Too much alcohol
  - Any alcohol during gout attacks
  - Foods and drinks sweetened with high-fructose corn syrup

It is to be kept in mind that just by modifying diet and avoiding purine-rich foods cannot solely prevent gout attacks. Medications are required for long durations to avoid sudden attacks of gout. As far as diet is concerned, a focus on maintaining an overall healthy weight, having a balanced diet, consuming sufficient fluids, and reducing alcohol consumption are all required to maintain normal physiological serum uric acid levels.

OTHER LIFESTYLE CHANGES TO HELP MANAGE AND PREVENT GOUT

Lifestyle changes that focus on physical activity and achieving and maintaining a healthy weight can also help to manage gout and keep it at bay if you do not have the condition. For those who do have gout, following your doctor's treatment plan will help keep your condition under control.

- *Lose weight*: Losing weight helps to decrease uric acid levels and the risk of gout attacks. Losing weight also reduces pressure on painful joints.

- *Get regular physical activity*: Regular physical activity can reduce uric acid levels. It also decreases the risk of obesity and other health conditions which can lead to gout formation. 150 minutes per week or more of moderate physical activity is recommended in adults.
- *Choose low-impact activities*: Moderate-intensity, low-impact activities such as walking, swimming, or biking put less stress on joints and make them less prone to injuries.

CONCLUSION

Effectively managing gout involves not only following beneficial practices but also avoiding triggers and behaviors that can exacerbate symptoms or increase the risk of gout attacks. By adhering to the "don'ts" outlined in this chapter, individuals with gout can minimize the severity and recurrence of their symptoms, improve joint health, and enhance their overall quality of life.

Managing gout requires a holistic approach that includes dietary modifications, lifestyle changes, and medication adherence. By following these do's and don'ts, individuals with gout can significantly improve their overall quality of life.

SUGGESTED READINGS

1. Neogi T. Clinical practice. Gout. N Eng J Med. 2011;364(5):443-52.
2. Choi HK, Curhan G. Obesity, weight change, hypertension, diuretic use, and risk of gout in men: the health professionals follow-up study. Arch Int Med. 2005;165(7):742-8.
3. Choi HK, Atkinson K, Karlson EW, Willett W, Curhan G. Alcohol intake and risk of incident gout in men: a prospective study. Lancet. 2004;363(9417):1277-81.
4. Perez-Ruiz F, Herrero-Beites AM. Evaluation of methods to measure serum urate in patients with gout: a systematic review. Rheumatology. 2008;48(8):155-7.
5. Becker MA, Jolly M. Hyperuricemia and gout. Mexdical Clin. 2006;90(4):549-60.

6. Zhang Y, Jordan JM. Epidemiology of osteoarthritis. Clin Geriatr Med. 2010;26(3):355-69.
7. Schlesinger N. Management of acute and chronic gouty arthritis: present state-of-the-art. Drugs. 2005;65(18):2425-41.
8. Dalbeth N, Haskard DO. Mechanisms of inflammation in gout. Rheumatology. 2005;44(9):1090-6.
9. Wallace KL, Riedel AA, Joseph-Ridge N, Wortmann R. Increasing prevalence of gout and hyperuricemia over 10 years among older adults in a managed care population. J Rheumatol. 2004;31(8):1582-7.
10. Tyson CC, Nwankwo C, Lin PH, Svetkey LP. The Dietary Approaches to Stop Hypertension (DASH) eating pattern in special populations. Curr Hypertens Rep. 2012;14(5):388-96.

CHAPTER **11**

Gout: The Unsatisfied Disease—A Complex Challenge in the Indian Scenario

Sachin Yashwant Kale, Arvind J Vatkar, Shivam Mehra

INTRODUCTION

Gout, an ailment as old as humanity itself, presents a paradox of medical intrigue and patient frustration. As an orthopedic surgeon with decades of experience, we have witnessed the myriad ways this disease intertwines with the lives of my patients, particularly in the Indian context. In this chapter, we shall delve into the perplexing issues of compliance, the recurrent nature of gout attacks, the scourge of alcohol addiction, and the elusive, shifting pains and swellings that confound both patients and physicians alike.

COMPLIANCE CONUNDRUM

Gout management, while seemingly straightforward with the advent of modern pharmacology, is beset with compliance challenges. The cornerstone of treatment lies in long-term urate-lowering therapy, predominantly with medications such as allopurinol or febuxostat. However, adherence to these medications is often inconsistent, leading to suboptimal control of the disease.

In India, several factors exacerbate this compliance issue. Socioeconomic constraints frequently impede regular access to medication. Furthermore, cultural beliefs and traditional medicine often clash with allopathic regimens, leading patients to abandon their prescribed treatments in favor of herbal remedies or other alternative therapies. Additionally, the asymptomatic periods between acute attacks foster a false sense of security, prompting patients to discontinue their medication, unaware that urate crystals continue to accumulate silently in their joints.

SPECTER OF RECURRENT ATTACKS

Gout's hallmark—sudden, excruciating attacks of arthritis—often recur with alarming regularity. These attacks are not merely painful; they are profoundly disruptive, impacting the patient's quality of life and productivity. In day-to-day practice, it has been seen how the fear of these unpredictable episodes looms large over patients, affecting their mental and emotional well-being.

Recurrent attacks are frequently precipitated by dietary indiscretions, dehydration, and, most notably, alcohol consumption. Despite comprehensive dietary counseling, the allure of purine-rich foods and alcohol remains a potent challenge, especially during social gatherings and festivals, which are abundant in Indian culture. The cycle of indulgence and subsequent agony creates a vicious loop that many patients find hard to escape.

ALCOHOL ADDICTION: A DUAL-EDGED SWORD

Alcohol, particularly beer and spirits, is a well-documented trigger for gout flares due to its high purine content and its ability to interfere with urate excretion. However, the problem is compounded when alcohol consumption crosses into addiction, a common issue in many parts of India.

Alcohol addiction not only exacerbates gout but also undermines the very foundation of patient compliance.

The intoxicating lure of alcohol can overpower the logical commitment to medication and dietary restrictions. This addiction often masks the underlying severity of the disease, leading patients into a dangerous complacency until a severe attack forces a painful reckoning.

ENIGMA OF VAGUE PAINS AND SHIFTING SWELLINGS

One of the most perplexing aspects of gout is the presentation of vague, migratory joint pains, and intermittent swellings. Unlike the classic acute monoarthritis of the big toe, these symptoms often do not fit neatly into the textbook description of gout, leading to diagnostic dilemmas.

In the Indian context, where access to advanced diagnostic facilities may be limited, these atypical presentations can lead to misdiagnosis or delayed diagnosis. Patients frequently visit multiple healthcare providers, receiving varying diagnoses such as rheumatoid arthritis, osteoarthritis, or even fibromyalgia, before gout is accurately identified. This diagnostic odyssey not only delays appropriate treatment but also adds to the patient's distress and dissatisfaction.

ADDRESSING THE CHALLENGES: A HOLISTIC APPROACH

Effective management of gout in India requires a holistic approach that transcends mere pharmacological intervention. Patient education is paramount. Empowering patients with knowledge about their disease, the importance of adherence to medication, and the role of lifestyle modifications can significantly enhance compliance.

Culturally sensitive dietary counseling is essential. Traditional Indian diets, rich in lentils, legumes, and certain vegetables, can be modified to reduce purine intake without completely overhauling the patient's culinary habits. Encouraging hydration and moderate exercise can further aid in preventing recurrent attacks.

Addressing alcohol addiction requires a multifaceted strategy, including psychological support, counseling, and, when necessary, pharmacotherapy. Integrating these services into routine gout management can help patients break free from the dual shackles of addiction and disease.

For those with vague and shifting pains, a high index of suspicion for gout should be maintained, and diagnostic efforts should include urate crystal analysis when feasible. Establishing dedicated gout clinics with access to ultrasound and dual-energy CT can improve diagnostic accuracy and patient outcomes.

CONCLUSION

Gout, with its recurrent attacks, compliance challenges, and the complicating factor of alcohol addiction, represents a multifaceted problem that demands a nuanced approach. In the Indian scenario, where cultural, socioeconomic, and healthcare accessibility issues intersect, managing gout becomes even more complex.

As healthcare providers, it is our duty to not only treat the disease but also to understand the lived experiences of our patients, guiding them through the labyrinth of symptoms, treatments, and lifestyle adjustments. Only through such comprehensive and compassionate care can we hope to tame this ancient, unsatisfied disease and restore our patients to a life of pain-free mobility and well-being.

SUGGESTED READINGS

1. Nieradko-Iwanicka B. The role of alcohol consumption in pathogenesis of gout. Critical reviews in food science and nutrition. 2022;62(25):7129-37.
2. Grassi W, De Angelis R. Clinical features of gout. Reumatismo. 2011;63(4):238-45.
3. Shiozawa A, Szabo SM, Bolzani A, Cheung A, Choi HK. Serum uric acid and the risk of incident and recurrent gout: a systematic review. The Journal of rheumatology. 2017;44(3):388-96.
4. Adamu SM, Akuyam SA. A Review of the Interactions Between Gout. BJMLS. 2018;3(1):94-103.

CHAPTER **12**

Topiroxostat, Febuxostat, Allopurinol, Colchicine, and Probenecid: A Review in Indian Communities

Bharat Veer Manchanda, Nindiya Kapoor Mehra, Shivam Mehra

INTRODUCTION

Hyperuricemia is caused by an increase in the levels of uric acid in blood. Elevation of serum uric acid (SUA) levels can be due to excess production or less excretion of uric acid. When SUA level is >6 mg/dL, it is termed as hyperuricemia.

Purine-rich foods (red meat, seafood, and beans) in the diet or high fat dairy products, drinks with added sugars, alcohol, or low secretion of uric acid due to kidney dysfunction and thiazide use and loop diuretics or physical activity in extreme are the main causes for increased production of SUA.

Gout is a type of arthritis in which a person experiences significant pain, stiffness, and edema in one or more joints. Dysfunction of purine metabolism is the main cause of this illness. There are several diagnostic possibilities, including a synovial fluid test, a uric acid blood test, and a differential diagnosis. Today, lifestyle changes and drugs are used as preventive strategies. In addition, gout is a disease that is frequently misdiagnosed as inflammatory arthritis. It is characterized by recurrent episodes of swelling, redness, and a sensitive, warm, and inflated appearance of the bone joint locations. The joints of the limbs, particularly the lower limbs, are affected, particularly the base section of the big toe and the first joint of the forefingers of the upper limbs. Tophus, urate nephropathy, and kidney stones are some of the major problems, which make life of patients miserable. Gout is caused by high amounts of uric acid in the blood over an extended period. When the concentration of uric acid rises too high, it crystallizes, and the crystals end up in the joints. As a result, the surrounding tissues are damaged, resulting in redness, edema, and inflammation, as well as a gout attack.

HYPERURICEMIA IN INDIA

Prevalence of hyperuricemia is around 25.8% in India. The occurrence of gout is more in males as compared to females, and it increases with age and ethnicity. Gout is still poorly managed in many nations, despite increased frequency and incidence. Urate-lowering therapy which is a definite, curative treatment is received by only a third to half of gout patients. The drugs used for gout and their mechanism of action are described ahead **(Flowchart 1)**. Fewer than half of these patients adhere to it due to adverse effects of conventional drugs. Obesity, nutritional variables, and comorbid conditions are all gout risk factors.

In addition to a well-established link between gout and an elevated risk of chronic kidney disease (CKD) and cardiovascular disease, new research has linked gout to atrial fibrillation, obstructive sleep apnea, erectile dysfunction, venous thromboembolism, and osteoporosis. Individuals with gout have been shown to have discrete patterns of comorbidity clustering.

Studies found that elevated uric acid levels are linked to metabolic syndrome laboratory and anthropometric markers.

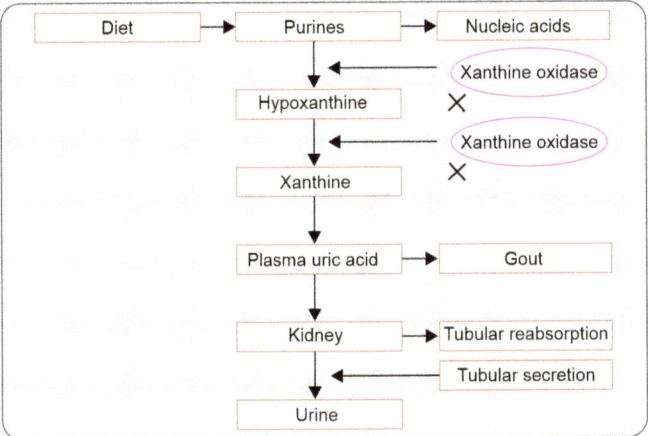

Flowchart 1: Basic mechanism of uric acid and drugs.

CLASSIFICATION OF ANTIGOUT DRUGS (FLOWCHART 2)

Based on Clinical

- Acute gout—colchicine, nonsteroidal anti-inflammatory drugs (NSAIDs), and steroids
- Chronic gout—allopurinol and probenecid

Based on Mechanism of Action

- Inhibit uric acid synthesis—allopurinol and febuxostat
- Increase uric acid excretion—probenecid
- Inhibit neutrophil migration into joint—colchicine
- Inhibit inflammation and pain—NSAIDs

Based on Nature

- Uricosuric—probenecid and sulfinpyrazone
- Uricostatic—topiroxostat, allopurinol, and febuxostat

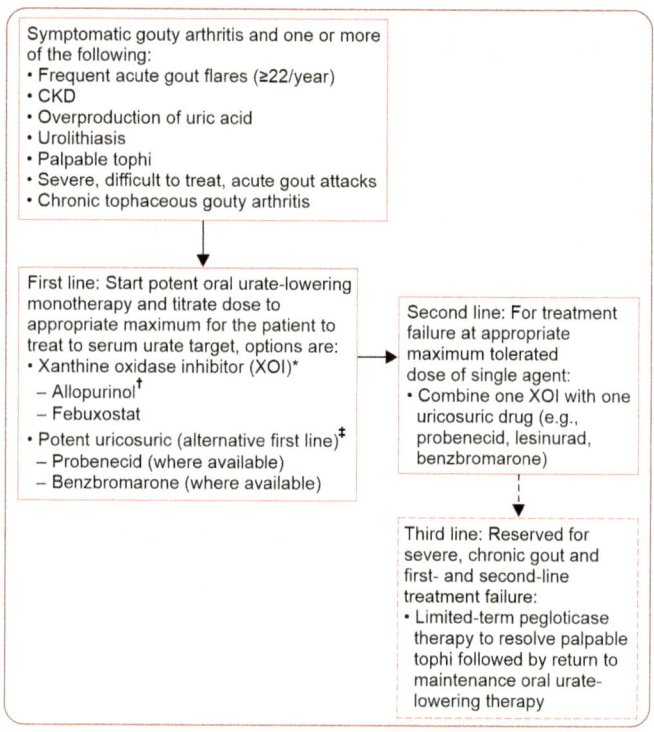

*Alternatives weighed by factors including cost of treatment, renal function and uric acid excretion, and drug tolerance.
†Prescreen for HLA-B*5801 by PCR-based test in populations at high risk of severe appopurinol hypersensitivity reaction [e.g., Han chinese, Thais, Koreans, Blacks (African descent)].
‡Requires renal function adequate for uricusouric response. Contraindicated with uric acid overproduction or urolithiasis.

Flowchart 2: Pharmacologic serum urate-lowering treatment.

(CKD: chronic kidney disease; HLA: human leukocyte antigen; PCR: polymerase chain reaction)
Source: Adapted from Hochberg MC, Silman AJ, Smolen JS, Weinblatt ME, Weisman MH, Gravallese EM. Management of Gout and Hyperuricemia. Rheumatology, 7th edition. Netherlands: Elsevier; 2018.

AIMS OF TREATMENT OF GOUT

The therapeutic aims in gout are as follows:
- To terminate the acute attack as promptly and gently as possible.
- To prevent recurrences of acute gouty arthritis.
- To prevent or reverse complications of the disease resulting from the deposition of sodium urate or uric acid crystals in joints, kidneys, or other sites.
- To prevent or reverse associated features of the illness that are deleterious, such as obesity, hypertriglyceridemia, and hypertension.

(*Source*: The aims of treatment of gout have been taken from the Kelly Textbook of Rheumatology, Gout and Hyperuricemia.)

TOPIROXOSTAT

Topiroxostat (nonpurine and xanthine oxidase inhibitor) inhibits the production of uric acid by suppressing both oxidized and reduced xanthine oxidase. Thus, it helps in managing hyperuricemia and gout.

Topiroxostat and its metabolites have been proven to be unaffected by renal impairment, suggesting that they could be useful for individuals with CKD. Topiroxostat does not have any adverse effect on the cardiovascular system and is safe to use.

Benefits of topiroxostat hyperuricemic drugs:
- A renoprotective drug
- Higher potential to lower lipid concentration
- Decreases microalbuminuria in diabetic patients
- Decreases urinary albumin creatinine ratio in CKD patients
- Cardiovascular safety

Mechanism of Inhibition

Topiroxostat has the strongest inhibitory action for the xanthine oxidase enzyme. Topiroxostat forms a reaction intermediate by forming a covalent bond with molybdenum, the reaction center of xanthine oxidoreductase (XOR), via an oxygen atom. It was also discovered that topiroxostat interacts with several XOR amino acid residues **(Flowchart 3 and Fig. 1)**.

Advantages of Topiroxostat over Other Antihyperuricemic Drugs

- Various clinical trials and papers based on clinical evidence have given a clear edge to topiroxostat in comparison to febuxostat and allopurinol in terms of safety and efficacy. There are very few adverse effects.
- Unlike traditional uricostatic medications, topiroxostat has a dual mode of action that provides patients with better and faster results.

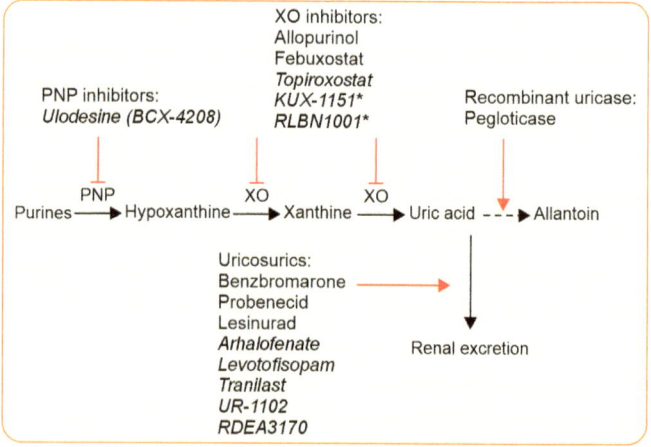

Flowchart 3: Mechanism of topiroxostat and other antigout drugs.

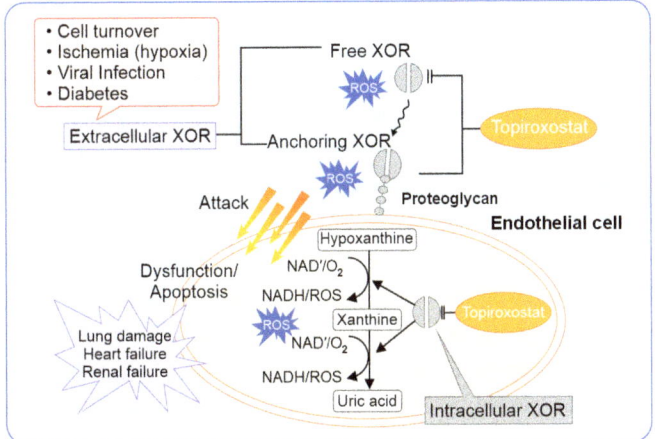

Fig. 1: Topiroxostat causes both intracellular as well as extracellular inhibition of xanthine oxidoreductase (XOR).

- Topiroxostat is a highly effective selective urate-lowering drug suggested to treat hyperuricemia.
- Topiroxostat is approved for use as a monotherapy in patients who are tolerating standard antihyperuricemia medications, as well as an add-on combination therapy when diet and exercise alone are insufficient to control hyperuricemia.
- Topiroxostat provides excellent urate-lowering management and lowers gouty flare and tophi formation across a broad spectrum of patients, according to clinical trials testing it as monotherapy and combination therapy.
- Superior hyperuricemic action of topiroxostat than febuxostat and allopurinol coupled with better safety profile makes it a better alternative to currently available anti-hyperuricemic drugs in India.

Indications
- Newly diagnosed hyperuricemic patients with or without gout
- Hyperuricemic patients not responding to conventional XOR inhibitors
- Hyperuricemic patients with comorbid conditions such as cardiovascular and renal patients profile

Adverse Reactions
- Nasopharyngitis
- Increased aspartate transaminase (AST) and alanine transaminase (ALT)
- Increased beta-2 microglobulin
- Increased blood creatine phosphokinase

Suggested Dosage
- *Initial dose*: 20 mg BD
- *Usual maintenance dose*: 40–60 mg BD
- *Maximum dose*: 80 mg BD

Review of Literature

An Indian study has been done in which they have taken multiple articles and they have reviewed all the articles very critically in which they have validated the efficacy of topiroxostat in managing hyperuricemia. The literature findings validate the safety, efficacy, and renoprotective effects conferred by topiroxostat, thereby corroborating its clinical use for reducing SUA level in patients with hyperuricemia. The positive effects of topiroxostat on renal function have been validated by almost all the studies considered in the review and its role in reducing SUA in hyperuricemia patients. Some of these major studies are ETUDE study, UPWARD study, TROFEO Trial, long-term multicenter, open-label study of topiroxostat by Hosoya et al., the study in hyperuricemic patients with CKD by Horino et al., and the study showing comparison of the effects of topiroxostat and febuxostat in patients with CKD.

Literature findings have also concluded on the low rate of serious adverse events with the majority of the effects being mild to moderate. The incidence of adverse events was comparable to that of allopurinol.

The study by Nakamura et al. has noted that the topiroxostat treatment promoted a dose-dependent reduction in the excretion of urinary albumin and plasma XOR activity. Similarly, a randomized, multicenter, double-blind study by Hosoya et al. noted that the therapeutic use of topiroxostat 160 mg in patients with hyperuricemia stage 3 CKD, irrespective of their gout status, helped in reducing urinary albumin excretion and SUA level. The study has also concluded on the concentration-dependent relationship between the efficacy of the drug in lowering serum urate and the drug safety. However, the low target SUA achievement rate (<50%) noted in the study may be due to a proportionally increased urate levels in the serum or deficit in the doses of topiroxostat. In a study by Katsuyama et al., topiroxostat reduced urinary protein and estimated glomerular filtration rate (eGFR) conferring renoprotective effects and reduced SUA level.

Majority of the studies have reported comparable efficacy of topiroxostat, allopurinol, and febuxostat. Hosoya et al. reported that topiroxostat and allopurinol had equivalent efficacy and no statistically significant difference in the occurrence of adverse events. Another study by Hosoya et al. noted that the efficacy of topiroxostat to lower serum urate levels is noninferior to serum allopurinol and both these drugs had comparable adverse events and drug reactions. According to Sakuma et al., the topiroxostat group had a significant reduction in uric acid levels at 24 weeks than the allopurinol group. In the cross-over clinical trial by Nagaoka et al., topiroxostat exhibited significant reduction in SUA levels and safety at the minimum dose compared to allopurinol. Sezai et al. reported that febuxostat therapy reduces serum urate level more dramatically and quickly than topiroxostat. However, there was no difference in serum urate levels between the two medications after 6 months and the efficacy was comparable. In terms of antioxidant activity, febuxostat outperformed topiroxostat after 3 months, but not after 6 months. Matsuo et al. reported comparable reduction in SUA level between topiroxostat and febuxostat. A study by Kario et al. found that topiroxostat and febuxostat were equally efficacious in decreasing SUA levels as there was no significant difference between the two and both the treatments were well tolerated.

Apart from the renoprotective and serum urate reduction benefits, the drug has been reported to confer cardiac safety.

There are several studies assessing the treatment of hyperuricemia with topiroxostat and with allopurinol or febuxostat. Uniformity in the ethnicity of the cohort considered in all the included studies is another advantage. The drawbacks of the included studies are lack of diversity, consideration of only the Japanese population, and not escalating the doses of allopurinol and febuxostat to the maximal level for attaining a reduction in SUA.

Miao et al. reported that the degree of reduction in serum urate level is linked to the long-term renal risk reduction. Correlation between the decrease of SUA levels and the increase in eGFR at 3 and 6 months after starting topiroxostat was reported by Katsuyama et al.

According to Mizukoshi et al., the antialbuminuric action of topiroxostat may not be dependent on serum urate levels. In the study by Kario et al., from baseline to 24 weeks, the urinary albumin-creatinine ratio decreased significantly with topiroxostat, but not with febuxostat. Whereas, serum urate levels decreased significantly from baseline in both the topiroxostat and febuxostat groups, implying that the antialbuminuric action may not be dependent on serum UA levels. According to Horino et al., the renoprotective effect of topiroxostat may be independent of its serum urate-lowering effect.

The present narrative review has significant relevance, as to the best of our knowledge, there is no review summarizing the clinical effects and safety of topiroxostat in managing hyperuricemia. Further, employing a more meticulous and prospectively defined objective process for the collection, extraction and compilation of data helped in the critical scrutiny of the study methodologies and excluding articles with unclear study designs and protocols and those not in the field of interest.

Conclusion

Topiroxostat can be considered as a safe and effective therapeutic choice for the management of hyperuricemia. The unique dual mechanism of action, cardiac safety, and renal protection are additional advantages of the drug in comparison to other currently available XOR inhibitors.

TREATMENT: THERAPIES FOR LOWERING URIC ACID

Indications

Candidates for uric acid-lowering therapy include patients who have multiple episodes of acute gout attacks per year or who have tophi on examination. To reduce the recurrence of gout attacks over time, reduce formation of tophi, and diminish the risk of joint destruction, uric acid lowering agents will be helpful. The indications for uric acid-lowering therapy are as follows:
- Tophi or chronic arthritis on examination
- Failure of colchicine prophylaxis of acute gouty arthritis
- Renal stones

- Prior to chemotherapy as prophylaxis of tumor lysis syndrome
- More than 12 mg/dL SUA levels which is extremely high.

Uric acid, formed at the end of purine metabolism (the nucleic acid component of DNA), is typically generated by the body during tissue restructuring and breakdown. Approximately, 20% of uric acid comes from purines consumed in food. Hyperuricemia has two main causes—(1) reduced elimination of uric acid by the kidneys and (2) heightened production of uric acid.

Reduced Renal Clearance (90% of the Patients)

- Kidney disease that originates within the organ itself.
- Heart conditions that result in reduced blood flow to the kidneys.
- Medications such as loop diuretics, low-dose aspirin, and cyclosporine
- Inherent genetic tendency
- Decline in glomerular filtration rate due to aging

Heightened Production of Uric Acid

- Unwise dietary choices
- Genetic predisposition
- Increased cell turnover due to tumors and lymphoproliferative disorders
- Stress-induced increase in adenosine triphosphate (ATP) turnover
- ATP turnover accelerated by alcohol consumption

Encourage all patients to adjust their lifestyle by reducing alcohol consumption, promoting weight loss when necessary, and reducing their intake of purine-rich foods. Additionally, it is important to manage any other medical conditions such as hypertension, diabetes, and high cholesterol.

List of Foods High in Purines

- High purine content—herring, mussels, yeast, smelt, sardines, and sweetbreads
- Moderate purine content—anchovies, grouse, mutton, veal, bacon, liver salmon, turkey, kidneys, partridge, trout, goose, haddock, pheasant, and scallops

Treatment Options for Lowering Uric Acid Levels

Before starting any uric acid-lowering treatment, it is important to be aware that there is a risk of triggering a gout flare. Therefore, a plan for managing this should be in place. This can usually be avoided by administering prophylactic medications (such as steroids, colchicine, and NSAIDs) along with uric acid-lowering therapy.

Probenecid

Probenecid is suitable for patients with reduced uric acid clearance by the kidneys and normal renal function. Generally, it should be used cautiously in patients over 60. Probenecid works by inhibiting the reabsorption of uric acid in the kidney's proximal tubules. The initial dose is 500–1,000 mg daily, which can be increased to 1,500–2,000 mg as required. In some cases, higher doses may be necessary. It is important to encourage good oral hydration as probenecid may lead to the formation of renal stones. This medication is not recommended for patients with renal stones (including calcium and uric acid stones) or those with urate nephropathy. Inappropriate use of probenecid in patients with hyperuricemia caused by excessive uric acid production can result in renal stones and urate nephropathy.

- Uricosuric
- This type of medication reduces the reabsorption of uric acid at the proximal renal tubules.

- It is beneficial for patients with reduced renal clearance of uric acid and can be used if the creatinine clearance is >40 cc/min.
- A 24-hour urine test for uric acid levels below 800 mg/dL is necessary for using this medication.
- Uricosuric medication can be employed even in cases of renal failure, but it does come with an increased risk of renal stones.

Allopurinol

Allopurinol is a commonly used and well-tolerated medication that helps lower uric acid levels. It can be initiated at a low dose of 100 mg daily (100 mg every other day if kidney function is very low) and adjusted by 100 mg every 10–14 days until the desired uric acid level of 4–5 mg/dL is reached. It is important to monitor liver function, blood counts, and kidney function while taking allopurinol. Possible side effects include rash, liver problems, bone marrow suppression, and severe allergic reactions. Allopurinol can interact with other medications such as warfarin and theophylline, so it is important to monitor levels. It should not be used in patients taking azathioprine, 6-mercaptopurine, or cyclophosphamide due to the risk of bone marrow toxicity.

As a xanthine oxidase inhibitor, allopurinol prevents the production of uric acid and is useful for patients with both increased synthesis and decreased clearance of uric acid. It does not require a 24-hour urine sample and can be used in patients with kidney failure. Rare side effects include bone marrow suppression, liver problems, and allergic reactions.

Febuxostat

In 2009, the Food and Drug Administration (FDA) sanctioned the utilization of a new xanthine oxidase inhibitor known as febuxostat for managing hyperuricemia in gout. It has shown a reduction in SUA levels depending on the dosage (80 mg or 120 mg/day). Its effectiveness has been observed in gout patients with mild or moderate kidney impairment. However, it may lead to irregularities in liver function tests, so regular blood work monitoring is advised. Just like allopurinol, febuxostat can interact with azathioprine, 6-MP, and theophylline.

- Xanthine oxidase inhibitor
- Hinders the production of uric acid and can be beneficial for patients with both increased uric acid synthesis and decreased clearance.
- It is suitable for use in cases of mild-to-moderate renal impairment.
- Bone marrow suppression and liver damage are rare side effects associated with its use.

Pegloticase

Uricase is an enzyme found in most mammals that converts uric acid into a more soluble form called allantoin. However, humans and some primates lack this enzyme, leading to difficulties in making uric acid more soluble and resulting in gout. Pegloticase, a porcine uricase, is an FDA-approved treatment for gout in patients who have not responded to standard therapies. It is administered through intravenous infusion every 2 weeks and requires premedication to prevent allergic reactions. Patients with a history of cardiac issues should receive this treatment with caution. The following should be kept in mind.

- Pegylated porcine uricase is effective for patients with either excessive production or poor elimination of uric acid.
- It enhances the solubility of uric acid.
- Patients need to receive premedication before infusions and be closely monitored for allergic responses.
- It is important to be cautious when using this treatment in patients with known heart conditions.

LIMITATIONS OF CONVENTIONAL URICOSTATIC DRUGS

Today many therapy alternatives are now available, including the use of NSAIDs, colchicine, steroids, and other medications. Allopurinol and febuxostat are some of the most commonly used medications. These medications have some drawbacks, including an increase in gout attacks during the initial treatment, higher risk of serious heart and blood vessel issues, and the possibility of developing a skin rash. Despite the introduction of new gout treatments, achieving the optimal levels of uric acid in the blood remains a challenge.

The difficulty of gout treatment regimens and insufficient convenience of use drugs, which result in poor patient adherence to standard antigout medication, are major factors to uric acid level nonadherence.

Limitations of allopurinol involve hypersensitivity or intolerance, failure of allopurinol to normalize SUA level and very high doses of allopurinol (e.g., >800 mg/day) required normalizing SUA level. In patients with CKD, dose reduction is required if creatinine clearance is <10 mL/min. Hypersensitivity responses and Stevens–Johnson syndrome are the most common side effects, followed by rash, fever, hepatitis, progressive renal failure, and bone marrow suppression. Although allopurinol is a first-line therapy for hyperuricemia, it is frequently linked with side effects and unsuccessful in lowering uric acid levels when used according to approved dose regimens. Managing patients with renal impairment is a significant limitation with allopurinol therapy and necessitate dose decreases.

Febuxostat tablets have the potential to cause cardiac impairment, liver function abnormalities (e.g., elevation of transaminases), nausea, arthralgia, gastrointestinal discomfort and headaches, etc. All these factors cause lesser patient adherence **(Table 1)**.

Table 1: Comparison of antihyperuricemic drugs.

Parameter	Allopurinol	Probenecid	Colchicine	Febuxostat	Topiroxostat
Indication	For treatment and prophylaxis of gout (treatment of hyperuricemia associated with gout and certain types of kidney stones; Prevention of increased uric acid levels in patients undergoing chemotherapy)	Treatment of hyperuricemia associated with gout. Adjunct to penicillin therapy to prolong plasma levels of antibiotics	• Acute gout flare treatment • Prophylaxis of gout flares • Familial Mediterranean fever	Chronic management of hyperuricemia in adult patients with gout who have an inadequate response to a maximally titrated dose of allopurinol, who are intolerant to allopurinol, or for whom treatment with allopurinol is not advisable	Gout, hyperuricemia

Continued

Continued

Parameter	Allopurinol	Probenecid	Colchicine	Febuxostat	Topiroxostat
Mechanism of action	Inhibits xanthine oxidase, reducing the production of uric acid	Inhibits reabsorption of uric acid in the kidneys, increasing excretion	Inhibits microtubule polymerization, reducing inflammation, preventing activation, degranulation, and migration of neutrophils associated with mediating some gout symptoms	Selectively inhibits xanthine oxidase	Nonpurine analog. Inhibits xanthine oxidase, reducing uric acid production
Doses	• Initial: 100 mg/day • Maintenance 200–300 mg/day (mild pour), 400–600 mg/day (severe 800 mg/day)	• Initial: 250 mg twice daily • Maintenance: 500 mg twice daily • Maximum: 2 g/day	• Acute gout 1.2 mg at the first sign of flare, followed by 0.6 mg 1 hour later (maximum 1.8 mg in 1 hour) • Prophylaxis: 0.6 mg once or twice daily	• Initial: 46 mg/day • Maintenance: 40–50 mg/day • Maximum: 120 mg/day	• Initial: 20 mg twice daily • Maintenance 40–60 mg twice daily

Continued

Continued

Parameter	Allopurinol	Probenecid	Colchicine	Febuxostat	Topiroxostat
Contraindications	Hypersensitivity to allopurinol HLA-B*5801 positive patients in patients of Korean descent with chronic kidney disease stage 3 or worse, or in patients of Han Chinese or Thai descent irrespective of renal function, is an especially high risk of AHS (allopurinol hypersensitivity syndrome) (higher risk of severe skin reactions)	• Hypersensitivity to drug • Blood dyscrasias uric acid stones • Children < 2 years of age • Coadministration with salicylates	• Severe renal or hepatic impairment • Concomitant use with strong CYP3A4 or P-gp inhibitors in patients with renal or hepatic impairment	• Severe hepatic impairment • Patients using azathioprine or mercaptopurine • Hypersensitivity to febuxostat	• Hypersensitivity to topiroxostat • Patients receiving mercaptopurine hydrate of azathioprine

Continued

Continued

Parameter	Allopurinol	Probenecid	Colchicine	Febuxostat	Topiroxostat
Renal safety	• Dose adjustment required in renal impairment • Risk of accumulation and toxicity if not adjusted	• Ineffective in patients with renal impairment (creatinine clearance <30 mL/min) • Increases risk of uric acid stones	• Dose reduction required in real impairment • Risk of toxicity in renal failure	• No dose adjustment for mild-to-moderate impairment renal impairment • Caution in severe renal impairment	Can be used in mild-to-moderate renal impairment with dose adjustments, pharmacokinetics of neither unchanged topiroxostat nor of its metabolites is affected by mild-to-moderate renal impairment

Continued

Continued

Parameter	Allopurinol	Probenecid	Colchicine	Febuxostat	Topiroxostat
Cardiac safety	Generally safe but rare reports of cardiovascular side effects (incidence < 1%)	Generally safe [probenecid appears to be associated with a modestly decreased risk of cardiovascular (CV) events including MI, stroke, and HF exacerbation compared with allopurinol]	Generally safe but caution advised in elderly patients or those with cardiac disease	Associated with increased risk of cardiovascular events (FDA warning)—in a CV outcomes shady, there was a higher rate of CV death in patients treated with Febuxostat compared to allopurinol, in the same study Febuxostat was noninferior to allopurinol for the primary endpoint of major adverse cardiovascular events (MACE). Consider the risks and benefits of Febuxostat when deciding to prescribe	Limited data, but generally considered safe (there have been no reports indicating the adverse effects of topiroxostat on the cardiovascular system)

CONCLUSION

The comparative analysis of topiroxostat, febuxostat, allopurinol, colchicine, and probenecid within Indian communities reveals the complexities involved in managing hyperuricemia and gout. Each drug offers distinct mechanisms of action, with topiroxostat and febuxostat serving as xanthine oxidase inhibitors, allopurinol as the traditional option with a well-established safety profile, colchicine as an anti-inflammatory agent for acute gout flares, and probenecid as a uricosuric agent promoting uric acid excretion.

In Indian settings, factors such as genetic predisposition, dietary habits, and socioeconomic conditions play significant roles in drug efficacy and safety profiles. Febuxostat and topiroxostat have shown promise in patients who are intolerant to allopurinol, while colchicine remains crucial for managing acute attacks.

Probenecid's utility, though limited due to its side-effect profile, can be beneficial in specific cases where urate lowering is insufficient.

Future research should focus on personalized medicine approaches, considering the genetic variability and specific risk factors prevalent in Indian communities, to optimize gout management and improve patient outcomes.

SUGGESTED READINGS

1. Ruoff G, Edwards NL. Overview of serum uric acid treatment targets in gout: Why less than 6 mg/dL? Postgrad Med. 2016;128(7):706-15.
2. Ragab G, Elshahaly M, Bardin T. Gout: An old disease in new perspective—A review. J Adv Res. 2017;8(5):495-511.
3. Billa G, Dargad R, Mehta A. Prevalence of hyperuricemia in Indian subjects attending hyperuricemia screening programs-a retrospective study. J Assoc Physicians India. 2018;66:43-6.

4. Dehlin M, Jacobsson L, Roddy E. Global epidemiology of gout: prevalence, incidence, treatment patterns and risk factors. Nat Rev Rheumatol. 2020;16(7):380-90.
5. Jaffe DH, Klein AB, Benis A, Flores NM, Gabay H, Morlock R, et al. Incident gout and chronic Kidney Disease: Healthcare utilization and survival. BMC Rheumatol. 2019;3(1):11.
6. Kundu AK. Gout in Indian Scenario. Textb Kundu. 2010;7:443-8.
7. Sato T, Ashizawa N, Iwanaga T, Nakamura H, Matsumoto K, Inoue T, et al. Design, synthesis, and pharmacological and pharmacokinetic evaluation of 3-phenyl-5-pyridyl-1,2,4-triazole derivatives as xanthine oxidoreductase inhibitors. Bioorg Med Chem Lett. 2009;19:184-7.
8. Chen CJ, Lü JM, Yao Q. Hyperuricemia-related diseases and xanthine oxidoreductase (XOR) inhibitors: An overview. Med Sci Monit. 2016;22:2501-12.
9. Nakamura T, Murase T, Satoh E, Miyachi A, Ogawa N, Abe K, et al. The influence of albumin on the plasma xanthine oxidoreductase inhibitory activity of allopurinol, febuxostat and topiroxostat: Insight into extra-urate lowering effect. Integr Mol Med. 2019;6(3):1-7.
10. Sattui SE, Gaffo A. Treatment of hyperuricemia in gout: current therapeutic options, latest developments and clinical implications. [online] Available from https://www.researchgate.net/figure/Uric-acid-pathway-and-action-site-of-urate-lowering-therapies-Drugs-in-italics-are_fig1_301795809 [Last accessed, 2024].
11. Hosoya T, Ishikawa T, Ogawa Y, Sakamoto R, Ohashi T. Multicenter, open-label study of long-term topiroxostat (FYX-051) administration in Japanese hyperuricemic patients with or without gout. Clin Drug Investig. 2018;38:1135-43.
12. Wada T, Hosoya T, Honda D, Sakamoto R, Narita K, Sasaki T, et al. Uric acid-lowering and renoprotective effects of topiroxostat, a selective xanthine oxidoreductase inhibitor, in patients with diabetic nephropathy and hyperuricemia: A randomized, double-blind, placebo-controlled, parallel-group study (UPWARD study). Clin Exp Nephrol. 2018;22:860-70.
13. Horino T, Hatakeyama Y, Ichii O, Matsumoto T, Shimamura Y, Inoue K, et al. Effects of topiroxostat in hyperuricemic patients with chronic kidney disease. Clin Exp Nephrol. 2018;22:337-45.
14. Mizukoshi T, Kato S, Ando M, Sobajima H, Ohashi N, Naruse T, et al. Renoprotective effects of topiroxostat for hyperuricaemic

patients with overt diabetic nephropathy study (ETUDE study): A prospective, randomized, multicentre clinical trial. Nephrology (Carlton). 2018;23:1023-30.
15. Kario K, Nishizawa M, Kiuchi M, Kiyosue A, Tomita F, Ohtani H, et al. Comparative effects of topiroxostat and febuxostat on arterial properties in hypertensive patients with hyperuricemia. J Clin Hypertens (Greenwich). 2021;23:334-44.
16. Sezai A, Obata K, Abe K, Kanno S, Sekino H. Cross-over trial of febuxostat and topiroxostat for hyperuricemia with cardiovascular disease (TROFEO Trial). Circ J. 2017;81:1707-12.
17. Hosoya T, Sasaki T, Hashimoto H, Sakamoto R, Ohashi T. Clinical efficacy and safety of topiroxostat in Japanese male hyperuricemic patients with or without gout: An exploratory, phase 2a, multicentre, randomized, double-blind, placebo-controlled study. J Clin Pharm Ther. 2016;41:298-305.
18. Hosoya T, Sasaki T, Ohashi T. Clinical efficacy and safety of topiroxostat in Japanese hyperuricemic patients with or without gout: A randomized, double-blinded, controlled phase 2b study. Clin Rheumatol. 2017;36:649-56.
19. Hosoya T, Ogawa Y, Hashimoto H, Ohashi T, Sakamoto R. Comparison of topiroxostat and allopurinol in Japanese hyperuricemic patients with or without gout: A phase 3, multicentre, randomized, double-blind, double-dummy, active-controlled, parallel-group study. J Clin Pharm Ther. 2016;41:290-7.
20. Nakamura T, Murase T, Nampei M, Morimoto N, Ashizawa N, Iwanaga T, et al. Effects of topiroxostat and febuxostat on urinary albumin excretion and plasma xanthine oxidoreductase activity in db/db mice. Eur J Pharmacol. 2016;780:224-31.
21. Hosoya T, Ohno I, Nomura S, Hisatome I, Uchida S, Fujimori S, et al. Effects of topiroxostat on the serum urate levels and urinary albumin excretion in hyperuricemic stage 3 chronic kidney disease patients with or without gout. Clin Exp Nephrol. 2014;18:876-84.
22. Katsuyama H, Yanai H, Hakoshima M. Renoprotective effect of xanthine oxidase inhibitor, topiroxostat. J Clin Med Res. 2019;11:614-6.
23. Nagaoka Y, Tanaka Y, Yoshimoto H, Suzuki R, Ryu K, Ueda M, et al. The effect of small dose of topiroxostat on serum uric acid in patients receiving hemodialysis. Hemodial Int. 2018;22:388-93.
24. Burns CM, Wortmann RL. Gout therapeutics: New drugs for an old disease. Lancet. 2011;377(9760):165-77.

25. Beatriz Vargas-Santos A, Neogi T. Management of gout and hyperuricemia in CKD Am J Kidney Dis. 2017;70(3):422-39.
26. Badve SV, Pascoe EM, Tiku A, Boudville N, Brown FG, Cass A, et al. Effects of allopurinol on the progression of chronic kidney disease. N Engl J Med. 2020;382(26):2504-13.
27. Jung JY, Choi Y, Suh CH, Yoon D, Kim HA. Effect of fenofibrate on uric acid level in patients with gout. Sci Rep. 2018;8(1):1-9.
28. Vos T, Abajobir AA, Abate KH, Abbafati C, Abbas KM, Abd-Allah F, et al. Global, regional, and national incidence, prevalence, and years lived with disability for 328 diseases and injuries for 195 countries, 1990–2016: a systematic analysis for the Global Burden of Disease Study 2016. The Lancet. 2017;390(10100):1211-59.

Summary and Key Takeaways

Gout, once known as the "disease of kings and king of diseases", is among the most ubiquitous etiologies of chronic inflammatory arthritis. The etiology of gout is usually multifactorial, including genetic predisposition, medical comorbidities, and dietary factors. In rare cases, a single genetic defect may be responsible for causing gout, usually associated with other medical complications. Irrespective of the underlying trigger, the result involves elevated serum uric acid, which can manifest as clinical gout in certain individuals.

The prevalence of gout in India is around 0.5%. A study done on the rural population of Belagavi, India revealed an overall hyperuricemia prevalence of 32.7%. However, still in the Indian context, we have less data that clearly elucidates the prevalence of hyperuricemia and gout in different populations and regions of the country. Nonetheless, a large number of Indians suffer from hyperuricemia and gout as is seen in the clinics. These numbers continue to increase. Through multiple studies, it has been shown that serum uric acid levels and gout disposition differ as per different populations, geographies, gender, age, etc. However, negligible studies are done in the Indian context (one such study data shown in **Table 1**).

The global gout therapeutics market in 2023 was 2.6 billion USD and is expected to grow to 5.4 billion USD by 2032. Also, as per data, the Asia-Pacific market is the fastest to grow specially Japan, China, and India. This data suggests that there is an immediate need for studies that can identify the prevalence of hyperuricemia and gout in different regions, populations, communities, age groups, gender, etc., in the Indian context to have better treatment options.

Table 1: Relationship between hyperuricemia (HU) and age categories and gender in subjects with type 2 diabetes mellitus and hypertension.

Parameters	Total number of subjects	Number (%) of subjects with HU	p value
Age groups			
≤ 30 years	104	18 (17.3)	0.0075[1]
31–50 years	1,112	337 (30.3)	<0.0001[2]
>50 years	1,566	602 (38.4)	<0.0001[3]
Gender			0.02[4]
Males	2,207	736 (33.3)	
Females	575	221 (38.4)	

[1] Age category ≤ 30 years vs. 31–50 years; $p = 0.0075$
[2] Age category 31–50 years vs. >50 years, $p < 0.0001$
[3] Age category < 30 years vs. >50 years, $p < 0.0001$
[4] Males vs. females, $p = 0.02$

Note: The data in the table has been taken from a study done in the Indian subjects attending Hyperuricemia Screening Programs.

Source: Billa G, Dargad R, Mehta A. Prevalence of hyperuricemia in Indian subjects attending hyperuricemia screening programs-a retrospective study. J Assoc Physicians India. 2018;66(4):43-6.

Our study on different religious communities is one such example that shows uric acid levels are higher in Sikhs as compared to Hindus, Muslims, and Christians when multiple factors such as diet, lifestyle, alcohol use, and smoking are taken into consideration. There is a need for more such studies as gout as a disease is multifactorial and results and revelations in the Indian scenario may or may not align with previous studies done in the Western countries. This will help in better treatment options and improving quality of life of Indian gout patients.

This book is an attempt to highlight gout and its effects in the Indian context.

Index

Page numbers followed by *f* refer to figure, *fc* refer to flowchart, and *t* refer to table.

A

Achilles tendinitis 59*t*
Adenine 17*f*
  metabolism pathway 16
  nucleotide breakdown 16
Adenosine
  diphosphate 16
  monophosphate 16, 21*fc*
  triphosphate 16, 21*fc*
Alanine transaminase 108
Alcohol 53
  addiction 97
  consumption 53, 87
    chronic 54
    limiting 54
  dehydrogenase 21*fc*
  metabolism of 21*fc*
Allopurinol 89, 96, 101, 103, 109, 114, 117*t*-121*t*
Antidiuretic hormone 51
Antigout drugs
  classification of 103
  mechanism of 106*fc*
Antihypertensive drugs 75
Antihyperuricemic drugs 106, 117*t*
Antiinflammatory drugs 38, 45, 82, 87
Antioxidant activity 110
Aspartate transaminase, increased 108
Aspirin, high-dose 90
Attack
  nighttime 61
  recurrent 61, 97
    specter of 97

B

Back pain
  acute 80
  chronic 80
Beta-2 microglobulin, increased 108
Blood
  creatine phosphokinase, increased 108
  test 6, 75
  volume, increased 70
Bloodstream 15
Body mass index 39, 73
Bone density, decreased 79
Bursitis 59*t*

C

Caffeine, metabolism of 21*fc*
Calcium pyrophosphate deposition disease 8
Carbon 1
Cardiovascular disease 2
Cardiovascular safety 105
Catabolism 15
Cell turnover, increased 70

Chemical
  molecule 1
  substances 1
Coffee 87
Colchicine 7, 38, 81, 101, 103, 117t-121t
Cold
  packs 47
    use 45
  therapy 45, 46
    causes blood vessels 46
Coronary
  endothelial dysfunction 41
  heart disease 40
Corticosteroids 7, 38, 75, 81, 89
Crash diets 89
Crystal
  deposition 78
  solubility and activity 45
Crystallization 50
Culturally sensitive dietary counseling 99

D

Dairy products 54
Data disposition 28
Dataset, analysis 28
  demography of 29
Dehydration 51
Diabetes mellitus, type 2 128t
Diet 69, 74, 90
Dietary
  changes 37
  factors 78
  modifications 37, 65
Disease-modifying antirheumatic drug 60

E

Enhanced sensitivity 44
Estimated glomerular filtration rate 109

Estrogen
  and uric acid excretion 35
  depletion postmenopause 34
  levels 34f
  postmenopausal decline in 35
Excretion, decreased 78
Exercise regularly 87
Extracellular inhibition 107f

F

Fat dairy, low 38, 86
Febuxostat 89, 96, 101, 109, 110, 114, 116, 117t-121t
Fetal
  complications 76
  growth restriction 71, 73
Fever 61
Fish 90
Fluid accumulation 44
Foods, limit processed 90
Footwear adjustments 66
Frozen vegetables 47
Fructokinase catalyzes phosphorylation 20
Fructose, metabolism of 21fc
Fruits and vegetables 86, 91

G

Gestational
  diabetes 69, 73
  hypertension 73
Glomerular filtration 18
Glomerular filtration, increased 35
Gout 1, 2, 33, 43, 57, 90
  acute 6, 103
  affected joints 43
  alcohol 50
  attacks, recurrent nature of 96
  biochemical basis of 50
  causes of 5

chronic 103
cold therapy for 46, 47
culprit for 49
diagnosis of 6
dietary strategies for managing 54
do's and don'ts 85
effective management of 98
flares, acute 81
foods to eat and avoid with 92*f*
in heel and retrocalcaneal region 61*t*
  management strategies for 65*t*
in postmenopausal women 35, 37
in pregnancy 68
in spine 77
management of 7, 54, 93
manifestations 58
onset or exacerbation of 33
pain 44
  managing 45
postmenopause 33
prevalence of 127
prevent 93
proteins avoided 52
related heel pain, management of 58
retrocalcaneal pain 64*fc*
risk of 40, 53, 55
symptoms of 6
treatment of 7, 105
unsatisfied disease 96
ways of management of 58
Gouty arthritis 49
Guanine 17*f*
  conversion 16
  metabolism pathway 16
  nucleotide breakdown 16

H

Health implications, long-term 54
Healthy
  lifestyle 55
  weight, maintain 86
Heat 43
  therapy 43
Heel
  and retrocalcaneal
    area 57*f*
    pain, cause of 58, 62*fc*
  deep pain in 63
  pad syndrome 60
  pain 57, 58, 63
    causes of understanding 58
  spurs 59*t*
  stiffness in 63
Hemodynamic changes 70
Hormonal changes 35, 70
Hot fermentation, using 43
Human leukocyte antigen 104
Hydration 7, 38, 45, 55, 65, 74
Hydrogen 1
Hypertension 5, 128*t*
  chronic 69
Hyperuricemia 1, 2, 3, 15, 21*fc*, 30, 39*f*, 68, 77, 101, 102, 128*t*
  causes of 5
  diagnosis of 6
  disorder 19
  in pregnancy 71, 72, 72*f*
    management of 74
    mechanism of 70, 71
    prevalence and causes 69
  management and prevention of 37
  mechanisms linking 78
  metabolism 22*fc*, 23
  pathophysiology of 77

prevalence of 102
proper management of 10
risk factors for 35
symptoms of 69
understanding 68
Hyperuricemic 16, 108
Hypoxanthine metabolism 16

I

Ibuprofen 45
Ice
  bath 47
  therapy 65
Idiopathic retrocalcaneal pain 57
Inflammation
  increased 43, 44
  managing
Inflammatory
  arthritis 33, 43
  cascade 78
  markers 81
  mediators 70
  response 51
Inhibit uric acid synthesis 103
Inhibition, mechanism of 106
Inosine conversion 16
Insulin resistance 71, 73
  pregnancy-induced 71
Intervertebral disk degeneration 79
Intestinal excretion 19
Intestines 15
Intrauterine growth restriction 71, 72f

J

Joint
  damage 9
    potential for 44
  fluid test 6

K

Kidney 15
  damage 75
  disease 5
    chronic 73, 104
      elevated risk of 102
      worsening of 71
  filtration and reabsorption in 18
  function 38
    reduced 70
  injury, acute 72
    potential for 71
  stones 9

L

Lactate dehydrogenase 21fc
Lean meats and poultry 54, 91
Lifestyle
  and dietary changes 46
  modifications 7, 74, 82

M

Magnetic resonance imaging 60, 62
Malaise 61t
Massage 43
Mean serum uric acid levels 30
Menopause 33
  research studies on 38
  stages of 34f
Metabolic
  disorders 19
  rate, reduced 46
  syndrome 2, 37
Microalbuminuria 105
Monosodium urate crystals 2
  formation of 77
Muscle spasms, decreased 46

N

Nasopharyngitis 108
Neurological
  manifestations 79
  symptoms 80
Niacin 5
Nicotinamide adenine
  dinucleotide 21*fc*
Nitrogen 1
Nonsteroidal anti-inflammatory
  drug 7, 31, 45, 60, 62, 81, 103
Nucleic acid 78
Numbing effect 46

O

Obesity 5, 69
  related hyperuricemia 74
Optimize therapeutic strategies 83
Organ meats 88
Osteoarthritis symptoms 9
Oxidant-antioxidant paradox 20
Oxidative stress 70
Oxygen 1

P

Pain 73, 63
  increased 44
  potential for increased 44
  sudden onset of severe 61
Pegloticase 115
Pegylated porcine uricase 115
Pharmacologic serum urate,
  lowering treatment 104*fc*
Phosphorylation of fructose 20
Physical activity
  decreased 37
  regular 38, 94
Physical therapy 65, 82
Placental
  dysfunction 70
  factors 70
  insufficiency 71
Plantar fasciitis 59*t*
Polymerase chain reaction 104
Postmenopausal
  hormone 34, 40
  prevention and management of 39*f*
  women 40
Preeclampsia 69, 71, 72, 72*f*, 75
Prenatal care 75
Probenecid 101, 103, 113, 117*t*-121*t*
Protein
  animal versus plant 52
  plant-based 54
  rich foods 53
Pseudogout 8
  crystals in synovial fluid of 8*f*
Psychological support 99
Purine
  and synthesis 21, 23
  breakdown 15, 16, 21, 23, 85
  content 52
  diet, low 46, 86
  foods, high in 88, 113
  metabolism
    byproduct of 49
    leads 19
  moderating 54
  rich
    foods 5, 101
    meats 93
    seafood 93
  source of 15

Q

Quality of life 97

R

Rat bite erosions 7f
Reabsorption 18
   reduced 35
Red meat 88
Religion, data disposition for 26t
Renal
   clearance, decreased 70, 112
   dysfunction 69
   function 104
      decreased 36
   insufficiency 78
   urate production 5
Renoprotective drug 105
Rest and joint protection 65
Retrocalcaneal pain 58
   causes of 59t
   understanding 58
Rheumatoid arthritis 60
   symptoms 9

S

Seafood 88
Septic arthritis symptoms 9
Serum uric acid 19
   elevated risk of 101
   levels 81
Shellfish 90
Skin condition, monitor 47
Spinal disorders 78
   risk factors for 79
Spinal stiffness 80
Standard deviation 29
Stress
   fractures 60t
   reduce 89
Student's t-test 29
Study sample
   dietary habits of 28t, 28f
   gender of 27f, 27t
   in different religions 27f
   lifestyle of 28t, 29f
   mean serum uric acid of 30f
   religion of 26f
Swelling 6, 44, 61, 63
   shifting
Synovial fluid, analysis of 81

T

Tarsal tunnel syndrome 60
Temporary relief 44
Tenderness 61
Tingling pain in heel and arch 63
Tophi 9, 81
Topiroxostat 101, 105-107, 109, 117t-121t
   advantages of 106
   causes 107f
   hyperuricemic drugs 105
   mechanism of 106fc
   reduced urinary protein 109
Transporter 9 18

U

Urate-lowering therapy 7, 81, 87, 96
   long-term 96
Uric acid 1, 2, 14, 86
   and drugs, basic mechanism of 103fc
   colorimetric measurement of 29
   concentration of 20
   endogenous production of 21fc
   excretion 15, 17, 19, 18f, 23, 104
      decreased 51
   first discovered 1
   formation 15, 16
      pathway of 17f
   from xanthine 15

increased production of 70
levels 38
   cause uncontrolled 89
   effect on elevated 25
   factors affecting 3
   increase in incidence of 33
   monitor 87
   regulation of 15
   treatment options for lowering 113
lowering drugs 38, 45, 111
menopause on metabolism of 34
metabolism 14, 34, 35
   in menopausal women 36*fc*
   in the human body 14
   normal 21, 22*fc*
   steps in 16
molecular structure of 2*f*
prevalence of 30
production 86, 112
   and excretion 50
   increased 51
research studies on 38
treatment, therapies for lowering 111
Uricostatic 103
   drugs 106
      limitations of 116

Uricosuric 103, 113
   response 104
Urinary albumin creatinine, decreased 105
Urolithiasis 104*fc*

V

Vague pains, enigma of 98
Vasoconstriction 46
Vitamin C rich foods 88
Volume expansion 70

W

Weight
   gain 36
   lose 93
   management 38, 46, 65, 74

X

Xanthine
   from hypoxanthine 15
   metabolism 16
   oxidase 16
      oxidizes xanthine 15
   oxidoreductase 107*f*
      reaction center of 106

EU GSPR Authorised Reprsentative
Logos Europe, 9 rue Nicolas Poussin
1700, La Rochelle, France
Phone: +33 (0) 6 67 93 73 78
E-mail: contact@logoseurope.eu

www.ingramcontent.com/pod-product-compliance
Ingram Content Group UK Ltd.
Pitfield, Milton Keynes, MK11 3LW, UK
UKHW020230220426
5322IPUK00017B/250